Practical Psychiatry for Students and Trainees

This is a welcome addition to the literature for medical students, newly qualified doctors, and very early career psychiatrists. As well as covering basic key clinical skills and information in an accessible way it provides extremely useful material on professionalism and self-care. This will be invaluable to all doctors starting out and beginning to discover the complexity and rewarding field of psychiatry.

—Kate Lovett, Immediate Past Dean,
Royal College of Psychiatrists, UK

This is an excellent, highly practical book for both medical students and for doctors at the early stages of their postgraduate training in psychiatry. It provides a highly readable overview of the key clinical areas, with use of mnemonics and valuable practical tips such as how to set up the clinical interview and sample phrasing of difficult-to-ask questions. This is combined with relevant reference to the underlying phenomenology and the evidence base.

—Anne Doherty, Consultant Liaison Psychiatrist,
Editor in Chief, Books Programme,
Royal College of Psychiatrists, UK

Practical Psychiatry for Students and Trainees

Anne-Marie O'Dwyer, M.D., M. Ed., F.R.C.P.I., M.R.C.Psych.

Clinical Professor
Department of Psychiatry
Trinity College Dublin & Consultant Psychiatrist
Psychological Medicine Service
St James's Hospital
Republic of Ireland

Mariel Campion, MB, MScLHPE, MRCPsych,

Senior Registrar in Liaison Psychiatry
St James's Hospital and Clinical Lecturer in Psychiatry
Trinity College
Republic of Ireland

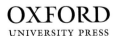

OXFORD
UNIVERSITY PRESS

OXFORD
UNIVERSITY PRESS

Great Clarendon Street, Oxford, OX2 6DP,
United Kingdom

Oxford University Press is a department of the University of Oxford.
It furthers the University's objective of excellence in research, scholarship,
and education by publishing worldwide. Oxford is a registered trade mark of
Oxford University Press in the UK and in certain other countries

© Oxford University Press 2022

The moral rights of the authors have been asserted

First Edition published in 2022

Impression: 1

Published in the United States of America by Oxford University Press
198 Madison Avenue, New York, NY 10016, United States of America

CIP data is on file at the Library of Congress

Data available

Library of Congress Control Number: 2021942158

ISBN 978–0–19–886713–5

DOI: 10.1093/med/9780198867135.001.0001

Printed and bound by
CPI Group (UK) Ltd, Croydon, CR0 4YY

This handbook is dedicated to our patients, from whom we learn our clinical skills. Their forbearance and kindness in allowing us to learn from them, often as they face extreme hardship in the context of illness, are simultaneously both humbling and heartening.

Our clinical skills are first laid down as students, often the most formative clinical learning experiences we have. The habits we learn then can persist for a lifetime. We owe it to our patients to start well.

Contents

Letter to the reader

Dear Reader,

Most students (especially medical students!) skip introductions. We hope that by speaking to you directly, we will stop your hand in mid-flight as it moves to 'skip' the introduction. While we initially wrote this handbook for medical students in psychiatry, it is for any of you unfamiliar with clinical interviewing. It provides students, and trainees, with core knowledge and the skills needed to deliver essential clinical care to patients with mental health needs.

The book places clinical interviewing skills—*what to ask and how to ask it*—and mental health in the context of medical (including Emergency Department and GP placements) as well as psychiatry settings. It considers the person within a global mental and physical framework. This reflects the authors' work as psychiatrists embedded in a general hospital, as well as clinical experience in medicine prior to psychiatry. Subsequent training with exceptional clinicians and teachers at the Maudsley and Institute of Psychiatry (London) and Addenbrooke's Hospital (Cambridge) for one of the authors (AMOD) provided formative clinical experiences in a true 'apprenticeship' style. The hope is to distil some of their clinical expertise and knowledge for future generations of students. This experience is combined with the practical approach and perspective of a psychiatrist approaching the end of comprehensive training as a junior hospital doctor (MC).

The handbook is an introduction to **practical clinical issues**. Each chapter outlines **key learning points**, **practical clinical tips**, and is illustrated with **clinical cases**. It provides specific guidance to enable clinicians to conduct a clinical interview with patients presenting with mental health needs. It also introduces core concepts of professionalism, burnout, and self-care, vital not only for the student clinician, but also for the patients whom they treat.

This is not a definitive textbook, nor is it a reference guide to research in psychiatry. It deliberately does not provide lists of references at the end of each chapter. It has not sought to include all areas. Instead, the text focuses on the more common issues that need to be grasped by the novice and, particularly, by students/graduates who may never again study psychiatry but will encounter mental health issues in all aspects of medical and surgical care. **Good clinical interview skills are essential for all clinicians** whatever their ultimate area of practice.

We assume no prior knowledge of psychiatry. The aim of the text is to be both clear and simple. The area of psychological ill-health and mental illness is, of course, neither clear nor simple. However, given that we remain almost exclusively reliant on our clinical skills and judgment, students should begin with a clear 'black-and-white' starting-point, from where they will then head into the multi-coloured reality of psychological disorders.

In writing any book in the modern age, one recognizes that rapidly advancing fields of technology render almost any textbook outdated on the date it is published. The fields of aetiology and treatments in mental health (and associated skills) are no exception. They advance and change rapidly each decade. This is in sharp contrast to skills required for human observation and assessment, which largely remain unchanged. Indeed, in medicine, clinical skills often decline with each decade, as students and doctors become more focused on technological examinations and interventions, than on the 'story' and observable findings in the person sitting in front of them. We hope that this book, with its focus on the clinical aspects of psychiatry, will go some way to address this imbalance.

How to use the book

The text is laid out in a specific sequence:

Section 1 (Chapters 1–4) presents important considerations in clinical interviewing: what to ask and how to ask it.

Section 2 (Chapters 5–10) presents common clinical conditions, starting with a chapter on personality disorders.

Section 3 (Chapters 11–15) presents some of the specialist areas: later life, child and adolescent, perinatal, intellectual disability, hospital and forensic psychiatry.

Section 4 (Chapters 16–18) focuses on management: how you should manage your patients, psychological therapies physical treatments, including medication and ECT, and emergencies.

The final section, Section 5, focuses on professionalism: how you should manage yourself.

Of necessity, there will be some overlap. This reflects the reality of mental illness as it presents. Thus, for example, suicide will be discussed in mood disorders, forensic psychiatry and in emergencies. Where possible, these cross-references are mentioned within the text.

While each chapter (and section) can be read on their own, they will probably be best understood if they are read in sequence.

It is the sincere hope of the authors that this text will encourage readers to delve further into the field of mental health. It is an on-going privilege to work in this area, challenging and rewarding in equal measure.

Professor Anne-Marie O'Dwyer MD, MEd, FRCPI, MRCPsych
Dr Mariel Campion MB, MScLHPE, MRCPsych

Acknowledgements

Many individuals have helped in this project, both directly and indirectly. It is inevitable that they will not all be individually named. We would like to thank them whole-heartedly for their encouragement and support.

The authors would like to specifically thank Professor Aiden Corvin, Head of Department, Psychiatry, Trinity College Dublin, for supporting the project both practically and academically.

Other colleagues, clinical academics who contribute to the teaching programme, generously donated their time to review sections of the book directed at their particular area of expertise. These include Sonya Collier, John Cooney, Philip Dodd, Conor Farren, Elaine Greene, Yvonne Hartnett, Eamon Keenan, Brendan Kelly, Harry Kennedy, Tara Kingston, Jasmin Lope, Simon McCarthy-Jones, Michael McDonough, Jane McGrath, Declan McLoughlin, Clare O'Toole, and Jamie Walsh. To those whom we have forgotten to include on this list we send a heart-felt apology. As busy clinicians, working in the realities of clinical practice, their experience makes their contribution to this practical clinical guide particularly valuable. Any remaining omissions, errors, or misconceptions are entirely the authors' responsibility.

A special word of thanks to Dr Lorna Power, doctor-in-training, former TCD medical student and talented illustrator, who has designed the cover.

Thank you also to Dr Eoin Kelleher, anaesthetist-in-training and accomplished cartoonist, www.eoinkelleher.com , who was commissioned to provide illustrations within the book.

Abbreviations

ACE	angiotensin converting enzyme
ACT	acceptance and commitment therapy
AD	Alzheimer's disease
ADHD	attention deficit hyperactivity disorder
AIMS	abnormal involuntary movement scale
AMT4	abbreviated-mental-test 4
AN	anorexia nervosa
ASD	autism spectrum disorders
BDD	body dysmorphic disorder
BDI	Beck depression inventory
BDZ	benzodiazepines
BMI	body mass index
BN	bulimia nervosa
BNF	British National Formulary
BP	blood pressure
BPAD	bipolar affective disorder
BPSD	behavioural and psychological symptoms of dementia
BPRS	brief psychiatric rating scale
BT	behavioural therapy
BZDs	benzodiazepines
CBT	cognitive behavioural therapy
CBT-E	enhanced cognitive behaviour therapy for eating disorders
CD	conduct disorder
CGI	clinical global impression
CK	creatine kinase
CRP	C-reactive protein
CT	computerized tomography
CVA	cerebro-vascular event
DA	dopaminergic
DASA	dynamic appraisal of situational aggression
DBT	dialectical behavioural therapy
DLB	dementia with Lewy bodies
DMV	diurnal mood variation
DSH	deliberate self-harm
DSM-5	Diagnostic and Statistical Manual of Mental Disorders

DST	dexamethasone suppression test
DZ	dizygotic
ECG	electrocardiogram
ECT	electro-convulsive therapy
ED	Emergency Department
EDDP	2-Ethylidene-1,5-dimethyl-3,3-diphenylpyrrolidine perchlorate
eGFR	estimated glomerular filtration rate
EMDR	eye-movement desensitization and reprocessing
EPSEs	extra-pyramidal side-effects
EUPD	emotionally unstable personality disorder
FBC	full blood count
GAD	generalized anxiety disorder
GAF	global assessment of functioning
GGT	gamma-glutamyl transferase
GHQ	general health questionnaire
HPA	hypothalamic–pituitary–adrenal
HR	heartrate
HVA	homovanillic acid
ICD-10	International Classification of Diseases
ICU	Intensive Care Unit
ID	intellectual disability
IDD	intellectual developmental disorders
IQ	intelligence quotient
LBW	low birth-weight
LFT	liver function test
MANTRA	Maudsley model of anorexia nervosa treatment for adults
MAOI	monoamine oxidase inhibitor
MaSSA	melatonin agonist and specific serotonin antagonist
MBSR	mindfulness-based stress reduction
MCV	mean corpuscular volume
MDT	multi-disciplinary team
MEN	multiple endocrine neoplasia
MI	myocardial infarct
MRI	magnetic resonance imaging
MSE	mental state examination
MSM	men who have sex with men
MZ	monozygotic
NAS	neonatal adaptation syndrome

NaSSA	noradrenergic and specific serotonergic anti-depressant
NATS	negative automatic thoughts
NES	non-epileptic seizures
NPS	new psycho-active substances
OCD	obsessive–compulsive disorder
OCP	oral contraceptive pill
OD	overdose
ODD	oppositional defiant disorder
OPD	Outpatient Department
OT	occupational therapist
OTC	over the counter
PANDAS	paediatric autoimmune neuropsychiatric disorders
PANSS	positive and negative symptoms of schizophrenia
PCL-R	psychopathy checklist-revised
PD	personality disorder
PDDs	pervasive development disorders
PDW	passive death wish
PND	postnatal depression
PO	per oram (by mouth)
PSD	post-stroke depression
PTSD	post-traumatic stress disorder
RFTs	renal function tests
SAD	somatoform autonomic dysfunction
SCID	structured clinical interview for DSM
SNRI	serotonin noradrenergic reuptake inhibitor
SSCM	specialist supportive clinical management
SSRI	serotonin specific reuptake inhibitor
TCADs	tricyclic anti-depressant drugs
TFTs	thyroid function tests
TNF	tumour necrosis factor
TSH	thoughts of self-harm
UEC	urea, electrolytes and creatinine

CHAPTER 1

The clinical interview—setting the scene

CHAPTER FOCUS

What you should know about the process of the clinical interview in psychiatry
- How to set up, safely and effectively, a clinical interview focused on mental health. The rationale for clinical interviewing in mental health.
- How to manage a clinical interview focused on mental health, particularly:
  - Safety.
  - Risk.
  - Rapport.
  - Opening, directing, and closing the interview, maintaining purpose and empathy.
  - Confidentiality.
  - Special circumstances.

1.1 Introduction—learning to drive

The diagnosis in psychiatry rests on the clinical interview. This is a practical skill. As with any practical skill, it requires knowledge and practice. Like the skill of learning to drive a car, initially every action must be carefully considered and planned. Rapidly shifting from one action to another is difficult. Then, with knowledge, practice, and experience comes confidence. The many components of the task become automatic, with an ability to 'shift gears' and 'alter direction' with ease.

Clinical interviewing is an integral part of all clinical medicine but is at its most challenging (and, arguably, most important) in psychiatry. Learning to interview forms the bedrock of practice, not only in psychiatry, but in all specialities, where most clinicians encounter patients with mental health issues.

1.2 Clinical interviewing: why do we do it?

In all clinical interactions, we should first ask ourselves: **what** we are doing and **why**? This ensures that we remain structured, focused, and logical.

We interview patients to:

- Gather information with a view to making a diagnosis.
- Develop a therapeutic relationship.
- Discuss diagnosis and management plans.

Of these, developing a therapeutic relationship is crucial, as without this, one cannot proceed. Components of clinical interviewing can mitigate against this: the need for exact information, lack of time, concerns about safety, all mitigate against a warm, empathic interview. These factors must be managed to optimize the therapeutic relationship within constraints.

1.3 What is needed?

Good clinical interviewing requires the ability to balance competing needs, the need to:

- **Control** the interview while maintaining **rapport**.
- **Manage** time while being **available** to (often distressed) patients.
- Ensure **safety** while promoting privacy/**confidentiality**.
- **Remember** key questions while **engaging** the patient.

Interview skills are best developed in their natural setting: observing experienced clinicians, noting their strategies (good and bad), interviewing patients oneself, getting feedback from others, and reflecting on the experiences. This is the aim of clinical attachments—**observe others and do it yourself**. To start this process, some **basic knowledge** is essential: the best format for the interview (see Chapters 2, 3); the terms used, the vocabulary of mental health (see Glossary); key strategies and tips for interviewing (provided throughout). This chapter focuses on key components in **setting up** the clinical interview: safety, risk, rapport, confidentiality, and special circumstances (Figure 1.1).

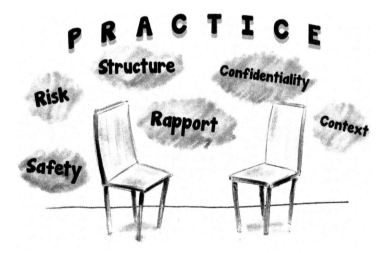

Figure 1.1 The clinical interview—setting the scene.
© Eoin Kelleher.

1.4 Safety first—the interview setting

Clinical vignette Interviewing in the Emergency Department (ED)

'Probably the most difficult issue in interviewing patients with mental illness in the Emergency Department is ensuring safety—for patients and staff. Patients are often agitated, distressed, unknown to us, and the environment can be chaotic. Safety is always my first concern. We cannot assess patients otherwise. I assume risk with every patient, implementing the same basic safety measures. This aims to both promote safety and reduce any sense of treating one cohort of patients differently. Everyone is treated with the same respect, care, and attention to detail.' Consultant in Emergency Medicine

People suffering psychological distress, if they do pose risk, are much more at risk of harming themselves than of harming others. However, a **small minority** pose a risk to others—staff and/or other patients. The best plan is **to promote safety at all times**. This maximizes safety, while minimizing any sense of stigmatization of one group of patients (see Clinical vignette Interviewing in the Emergency Department). The safety points below should be in place for all settings.

1.4.1 Key safety points

- **Inform** yourself about the patient **before the interview**—review with staff and (available) notes. *The best predictor of violence is past history of violence.*
- **Inform** staff members whom you are going to interview, and where.
- **Check** the interview room:
  - There should be two exit points—ensure exits are not locked/blocked beforehand.
  - If the room only has one exit, make sure the patient is not sitting between you and the exit.
  - If possible, review the room beforehand and remove all objects that could be used as weapons.
- **Sit,** and invite the patient to sit (can de-escalate a tense interview).
- **Leave** the interview if you feel at risk, or the situation is escalating beyond your control (see Table 1.1, Practical tip Interview Techniques Summary). Do not enter into further discussion. The clinician cannot help if they themselves are at risk (see Clinical vignette Safety: what not to do).
- **Ask** for a chaperone if you feel there is a risk of aggression—do not see the patient on your own.
- Have a **plan** to manage and contain the situation if it is likely that the patient may require emergency containment.

Table 1.1 Practical tip—interview techniques summary

Directing the interview	Questioning techniques	
I am sorry to stop you, but could I ask you about x as I am particularly concerned about that?	**Closed vs. open** *How are you feeling at the moment?* (open) *Is your mood good or bad?* (closed)	**Leading vs. non-directive** *Are you sleeping badly?* (leading) *Can you tell me about your sleep patterns?* (non-directive)
Thank you for that information, I will come back to that, but could I just focus for a moment on …?	**Managing sensitive disclosure or questions (for students)** *I can see this is very difficult for you and is very important. Some of what we discuss may have to be disclosed further. Is it okay if I ask to get my supervising doctor's advice?* *I am afraid I do not know the answer to that question. I am a student doctor with the team. Would you like me to discuss that with my supervising doctor?*	
How to leave an interview that is escalating while maintaining engagement*		
I appreciate that you are very upset. I need to ask for help so that I can help you with that. I will be back shortly.	* Or, where a person is not mentally ill but has become aggressive and hostile: *I am sorry I cannot continue the interview. I will be back shortly.*	
Ending the interview		
I am going to have to finish the interview in the next few minutes. Is there anything you would like to add, anything I should have asked about?	*I am going to say back to you what I think you have told me and what I have understood. If I get anything wrong, please correct me.* *Is there anything you would like to ask?*	

Clinical vignette Safety: what not to do

'I was a [young, slight, enthusiastic, female] junior doctor early in my training in mental health. I was on-call in a busy ED in central London. I was interviewing [on my own] a tall, well-built young man who was psychotic and agitated. He became more agitated as the interview progressed, saying he was hearing voices. He suddenly stood up and strode towards the [only] door of the interview room to leave. I was so intent on looking after him that I stepped forward to block his exit. Fortunately, he stepped around me but now stood between me and the only exit, distressed and shouting at me about the voices in his head that were tormenting him, asking if I were involved.' Consultant Psychiatrist

1.4.2 Clinical vignette Safety—what should have happened

If the junior doctor had used the safety points outlined in Key safety points, she would have:

- Been informed by staff and notes that the patient had a history of both psychosis and violence.
- Asked for team members to be with her for the interview.
- Planned for the potential need to escalate to rapid containment (by a team of staff), if needed.

Fortunately for the junior doctor, the patient (despite being distressed and un-well) did not harm her. Other staff members heard the noise and came to help. It was a valuable learning experience, but a potentially dangerous one. Please ensure that you put safety strategies in place **every time** you see a patient.

1.4.3 Safety—managing personal questions about you

The issue of managing personal interactions within a professional setting is a complex one, discussed further in Chapter 19. Every doctor has their own individual style—even an (apparently) simple concept of the use of first-name terms can lead to lively discussion. A 'safe' guideline for those early in their career (and, I would argue, throughout your career) is to be very clear in the boundary between personal and professional. This can be difficult when patients ask you apparently simple questions like: *Do you have children yourself?*. Refusing to answer this on the grounds of professionalism can seem insensitive, even rude. Yet decisions to share personal information must be taken very carefully, as their implications may range far beyond what you imagine. Some of your patients may be infertile and distressed about this, others may have had children who died, some may no longer have access to their children—so that these 'innocent' questions may colour and distort your relationship. In a forensic setting, interviewing someone with a history of violence, it is particularly unwise to share family details. You will need to consider your replies. A suggestion is to thank the patient for asking, pointing out that the interview is about them, not you, and reflecting the question back, e.g. *Thank you for asking, but this interview is focused on you not me—could you tell me more about your children?*.

1.5 **Risk**

The terms 'risk' and 'risk assessment' have crept into medical assessments, frequently included as 'boxes' to be 'ticked'. Yet, 'risk', by definition, refers to the future—the possibility/chance/likelihood of an adverse event. Doctors cannot predict the future. What we can do, however, is use assessment to identify factors that **increase the likelihood** of an adverse event (generally considered **risk of harm to self or others**) and consider **ways to mitigate** these factors. Psychiatrists should be particularly well-placed to help in the presence of an underlying mental illness (e.g. severe depression, psychosis). However, this is a very complex area and the relationship with mental illness is not always clear. Furthermore, as with safety, in clinical practice, 'risk' for the patient (of harm to self or others) should be considered at **every point** of the interaction. In this handbook, therefore, 'risk' is embedded throughout—in assessment, examination (see Chapters 2, 3), and in chapters on mental illness and emergencies. Please refer to Chapter 15 for detailed discussion and consideration of this complex area.

1.6 Rapport

Once you have confirmed that your environment is safe, the next step is to promote rapport. This is a difficult balance between empathy, engagement, listening with safety, time-limits, and control (see Clinical vignette Rapport). It is equally important to consider things that may be unhelpful for rapport (see Practical tips Rapport—things NOT to say or do at clinical interview).

Clinical vignette Rapport

'It is an irony that we must build rapport, establish a safe, confiding relationship, in a busy hospital environment, where so many factors mitigate against that—no privacy, no time, concerns about safety. I have learned to use key items to build rapport whatever the environment, to give the message to the patient that they are the only important person for me at that moment in time. How do I do that? Having introduced anyone who is with me to the patient, I then try to block out everything around us, focusing only on the patient, sitting down (even on a busy hospital ward) to be at their eye-level, to give the message that I have time. It is difficult, but small things convey that I am there to hear their story.' Medical Consultant

'I have learned to intervene early if I think the patient is going to disclose something I may be obliged to reveal as it can be so damaging for the therapeutic relationship. I have key phrases I have developed: "I can see that you are very distressed about this and am very glad that you feel able to discuss it with me. As you know, our conversations are entirely confidential. But there are some cases where I must inform others (perhaps a social worker or members of the police) if there is a risk of harm to someone else."' Consultant Psychotherapist

---

1.6.1 Opening the interview

- **Introduce** yourself and anyone with you, explaining their role.
- **Confirm** that they are willing to see you.
- **Sit down:**
  o At an appropriate distance (not too close).
  o Ideally, without a large desk between you.

○ At an angle to the patient, so that you are not facing 'head-to head' (allows the patient to break eye-contact, if needed).

○ To be at eye-level with the patient (standing 'towering' over a patient can be very intimidating).

- **Indicate** (if possible) the time you are likely to spend.
- **Check** if they have a relative with them and whether they are willing for you to speak to the relative for collateral history (supporting history from someone close to them).

1.6.2 During the interview

- Maintain good **eye contact** and focus on the patient.
- Keep note-writing to a minimum and reduce the intrusion by 'normalizing' it with the patient with a statement, e.g. *Apologies that I am taking notes, but it helps me to ensure I remember all the information. If you are bothered by it or have questions please let me know.*
- Allow time to **listen**—initially let the patient speak without interruption.
- **Repeating** phrases the patient has used shows you have been listening and is useful for prompting more information. Some phrases can be used in any situation:
  ○ *It was frightening? You were anxious?*
  ○ *Can you tell me more about that?* (a particularly useful generic question).
- **Control** the interview while remaining respectful of the patient's needs, e.g.:
  ○ *Thank you for telling me that. I can see it was very important to you—I will come back to it. But could I just focus for a moment on your mood?*
  ○ *Could I just interrupt you briefly to ask how you were sleeping?*
- Do not leave '**difficult/upsetting**' questions to the end of the interview. Address them during the interview, as ending the interview well requires particular skills (see the following section).

1.6.3 Closing the interview

Drawing an interview to a close can be very difficult, especially if you are short of time and the patient feels they still have things to discuss. The following are some points that can help to end an interview respectfully:

- **Indicate** that the interview is coming to an end:
  ○ *I am going to have to end this interview in a few minutes time.*
- **Summarize** what they have said:
  ○ *I am going to summarize what you have told me. Can you correct anything I have gotten wrong or have omitted?*
- **Give** the patient an opportunity to say anything else that is important:
  ○ *I will have to end this interview in a few minutes time, is there anything else you need to add or ask?*

- **Offer** another time, if that is needed (and possible):
  - ○ *I am going to have to end this interview in a few minutes. I can see there are other things you would like to discuss, would you like to arrange another time to meet?*
- **Ask** if they have any other questions and/or anything they need to add, while still being clear that you have to end the interview in a few minutes. **Wait** for their answer. If they add something long, complex, and new, an example of what you can say is:
  - ○ *Thank you for telling me that. I can see you have more to say about it. As I have said, I need to end this interview in a few minutes, so perhaps we can arrange to meet again to discuss that.*
  - ○ Or if you are a student and unlikely to meet the person again: *Thank you for telling me that. I can see you have more to say. As I have said, I need to end this interview in a few minutes, and, as you know, I am a student—would it be okay if I told a team member so they can discuss it further with you?*

1.6.4 Ending the interview

- **Thank** the patient for their time.
- **Indicate** what the next step is:
  - ○ *Thank you for your time. It was very helpful for me. I am going to speak to other members of the team, as we discussed.*
- **Escort** the patient to the door and ensure they know their way out.

Practical tips Rapport—things NOT to say or do at clinical interview

Key phrases and behaviours that can be very unhelpful:

- 'I understand'—many patients feel you cannot possibly understand, particularly in your first interview as a student.
- 'I'm sure it will be fine'—patients do not appreciate premature or uninformed reassurance.
- 'If you can just calm down'—generally causes an escalation in anger.
- Sneaking glances at one's watch—patients are (understandably) acutely aware of all our behaviours during an interview. They will notice and will (rightly) assume it is a sign of lack of engagement with the interview process. If stuck for time, please see the suggestions above for helpful phrases.
- Checking one's mobile phone—should be switched off. If, for some emergency, you must be available, tell the patient at the start of the interview and explain why. Apologize if, in those circumstances, you have to answer it.
- Reading through the patient's notes while they wait—should be done before the interview.

1.7 Confidentiality

Patients' information is **always** confidential to their doctor, except in a small number of specific instances. The nature of a psychiatric interview means the person is disclosing particularly sensitive information. For the most part, information is **not shared** without the individual's consent. There are exceptions (please see Practical tips Confidentiality).

1.7.1 Breaching confidentiality:

Information cannot be disclosed to third parties without consent with some specific exceptions. Examples include:

- Risk of serious harm or death:
  - ○ Specific threat to harm someone—duty of care to warn that person (Tarasoff doctrine).
  - ○ Suspected child abuse—where patient discloses details of the alleged abuser.*
  - ○ Risk of harm to the public (e.g. continuing to drive while unsafe).
- Specific legal instances where information must be shared:
  - ○ Public health/communicable disease.
  - ○ Request from a court (information immediately relevant to the enquiry).
  - ○ Interviews for specific purposes (e.g. preparation of a court report in respect of an alleged offence).

*In many countries, e.g. Children's First Guidelines (Republic of Ireland) (www. dcya.gov.ie), there is a mandatory duty to report any disclosure of childhood abuse—even if the patient does not give consent. The perpetrator may still be alive and, therefore, poses an ongoing risk to other children. Please check guidelines in your jurisdiction.

These are very serious issues. If they do arise:

- Ensure that a breach in confidentiality will, in fact, be required (consult with a senior team member).
- Disclose to the minimum number of people and ensure they understand their own duty of confidentiality.
- Inform the patient about the need to breach confidentiality (unless to do so would have other consequences, e.g. risk of harm to others).

As with mental health legislation, you will need to consult your local jurisdiction for more detailed guidance (e.g. the Medical Council). These are always difficult situations—**always consult colleagues for advice.**

These issues are even more complex for **students** who should probably intervene early to ensure that someone more senior can be involved, using the example above, but modifying it: *I can see that you are very distressed about this and am very glad that you feel able to discuss it with me. However, as you know,*

I am a student attached to this team and think it would be far better for someone more senior in the team to discuss this with you. I can ask them to come to see you—is that okay?

Practical tips Confidentiality

It can be extremely difficult if one must breach confidentiality, as it can harm the relationship. To minimize the risks:

- Be well-informed of the above instances.
- Discuss with the patient early in the interview, if needed.
- Have a strategy to manage the situation, if it arises.

1.8 Special circumstances

Always be aware of the impact of **cultural differences** (see also Chapter 2):

- The stigma of mental illness is greater in some cultures than in others. This may impact on willingness to volunteer information or to accept treatment.
- Events deemed stressful differ between cultures.
- In some cultures, distress is expressed through **physical** symptoms.
- What is considered to be a normal expression of distress in one culture, may be perceived as illness in another.
- Beliefs considered 'normal' in one culture, may be misdiagnosed as delusions by an interviewer unfamiliar with cultural norms.
- Talking to family, where possible, and sourcing an interpreter of the same cultural background as the patient is helpful.

The interview is made even more difficult if an **interpreter** is needed. Please be aware that an interpreter, if needed:

- Must **directly translate**, not paraphrase, what the patient says.
- Despite speaking the same language, may not have the same cultural background.
- In some cultures, differences in gender may be problematic.
- Will necessarily require more time.
- Increases difficulty in establishing rapport.

Extra detail on other specific cases is available in the relevant chapters, for example, Chapters 11 and 12. See Table 1.1 for a summary of interview techniques.

1.9 Summary

Interviewing is a **key skill** for all clinicians. It is the cornerstone for the therapeutic alliance. Learning to do it well is helped by learning key phrases and behaviours, using tips and strategies, and **practice**. It is immediately clear to patients and colleagues (and examiners) whether a student is familiar and comfortable with the interviewing process—practice, practice, and practice. This chapter has provided information on how to set up and manage a clinical interview—**how to ask**. The following chapters provide the detail on **what to ask**—the history and examination.

CHAPTER 2

The psychiatric history— what to ask

What you should know about taking a psychiatric history—'what to ask'

- The **structure** and **headings** of the psychiatric history.
- **Key questions** to ask in each section.
- How to **follow clues** to **expand** on information presented.
- **Specific** examples for 'what to ask' in sensitive areas.

2.1 Introduction—learning to drive

Continuing the analogy from Chapter 1, knowing a specific structure for the psychiatric history helps the process to become almost automatic, allowing you to naturally respond to cues from the patient, promoting rapport. This chapter sets out a structure and headings that are useful for the task. The process is similar to a 'medical' history where one uses the person's **own terms** for the **history**, and **'medical'** terms (**psychopathology** terms in mental health) when presenting the **examination**. As with medicine, it is important to be familiar with these terms and their exact meaning (see Glossary). Thus, for example 'feeling breathless when they exercise' in a patient with signs of pneumonia on examination may be presented as 'a history of dyspnoea on exertion with signs of consolidation bibasally'. In mental health 'hearing voices, which he believes are real, talking about him', may be presented as 'agitated with third-person commentary auditory hallucinations to which they responded during the interview'. Much of the skill in history-taking is in following the 'clues' that the patient presents, making a hypothesis of what might be the underlying cause, and searching for evidence to support or refute that hypothesis (Figure 2.1).

Thus, the **psychiatric assessment** requires **knowledge** of:

- How to **set up** and **manage** a clinical interview (see Chapter 1).
- Specific **terminology** (see Glossary).
- A logical **structure** (key headings) for the patient's **history** (this chapter) and **examination** (see Chapter 3).
- **Symptoms** and **signs** of mental illness (chapters relevant to specific symptoms and signs throughout the book).

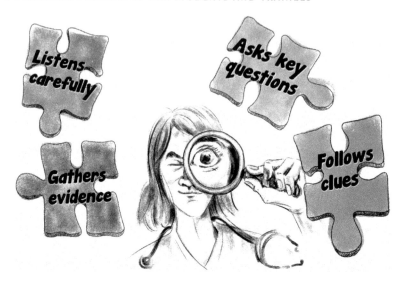

Figure 2.1 Taking a history—be a detective.
© Eoin Kelleher.

2.2 Key headings in psychiatric history

The psychiatry history follows a logical format, using a set of key headings (see Box 2.1 and Practical tips History-taking—how to 'remember' the headings) which act as:

- **Prompts** to remember key areas about which to ask.
- **'Anchors'** to provide structure.
- **Framework** to understand presentation and aetiology.

Practical tips History-taking—how to 'remember' the headings

- Taking a history is a logical process. One doesn't need a mnemonic to remember the headings. Simply follow the person's life-course and the headings become automatic, e.g. birth, early childhood, school, etc.
- Always consider **why** you are asking a question—how can the information help you understand the presentation—this helps to structure your history.

Box 2.1 Key headings in psychiatric history

Introduction
Presenting complaint
Past psychiatric history
Past medical/surgical history
Family history
Personal history
Substance use, medication, allergies
Current social/specific circumstances
Forensic history
Premorbid personality

2.2.1 Introduction

This includes basic demographic information (age, marital status, occupation, context of referral):

> *Mr X, a 46-year-old married father of two, an accountant, was referred to out-patients by his GP for assessment of mood.*

2.2.2 Presenting complaint

- The patient's concerns in their own words (specific quotes are useful) (see Practical tips Presenting complaint—be a 'detective').

2.2.2.1 History of presenting complaint

A logical expansion on the presenting symptoms:

- **When** they started.
- **What** was happening when they started (possible stressors).
- **What** makes them worse/better.
- Have they **changed** over time?
- **Impact** on the person's life:
  ○ Work, relationships (i.e. functional impairment).
- **Effect** of any intervention.

Practical tips Presenting complaint—be a 'detective'

- The initial presenting complaints are '**clues**' as to what might be behind the presentation, e.g. 'feeling low, no interest' suggest depression.

continued >

- The history of the presenting complaint is then your efforts to search for 'evidence' that supports or refutes the suggested diagnosis. So, for example, for depression, you would then search for history of reduced pleasure, early morning wakening, and other symptoms whose presence support that diagnosis. If they are absent, the diagnosis is much less likely. You need to search in a different direction.
- Patients will not be able to discern which symptoms are relevant, so you must **sift** through information presented and highlight **relevant** findings— the 'evidence'.

Clearly, this specific process requires **knowledge** of the main conditions (you will learn this from later chapters). Examples include:

- The **absence** of symptoms that one would expect to find, e.g. no sleep or appetite disturbance in someone presenting with depressive symptoms.
- The **presence** of symptoms that suggest severity of the illness, e.g. psychotic symptoms in depression, command hallucinations in psychosis.

2.2.2.2 Deliberate self-harm (DSH)

Concern about suicide (and self-harm), permeates all psychiatry assessments— the focus is guided by the presenting complaint. Thus, for example, in depression, it is likely to form part of the presenting complaint assessment. In other presentations, it may be 'screened for' in the mental state examination or it may be introduced within past history, with a history of previous self-harm. It is such an important topic that you will find it cross-referenced in several chapters in this handbook (see Chapters 3, 6, 15, and 18).

What and how to ask in this area are presented here, although, as noted, they may present more naturally in the past psychiatric history or the mental state examination, depending on the patient.

2.2.2.3 Specific thoughts about self-harm or suicide

- Asking about self-harm/suicide does not increase the risk of someone acting on such thoughts.
- It is an **essential** part of any history—always ask about it. You should have a structure for doing this (see Table 2.1 for useful questions, placed on spectrum of severity).
- There may be a sense of relief at being given an opportunity to discuss these thoughts.
- Thoughts of self-harm or suicide **exist on a spectrum of increasing severity/risk:**
  ○ Passive death wish (PDW)—the individual feels they would be better off dead/not being alive but they have made no active plans to harm themselves.

Table 2.1 DSH useful questions

Questions		Place on 'spectrum' of TSH*
Have you ever felt it was too difficult to go on, as if life was not worth living? Did you ever go to bed at night and not care if you didn't wake up the next morning?	I N C R E A S I N G S E V E R I T Y	Passive death wish (PDW)
(If yes) have you ever considered doing anything about this/harming yourself?		Thoughts of self-harm (TSH)
(If yes) have you any specific plans? Can you tell me more? Have you acted on those plans/have access to these means? (particularly important with violent means, e.g. shotguns)		Plans for suicide
(If yes), do you intend to act on this? When?		Suicidal intent
Have you done anything specific (e.g. made a will, given away pets)?		Final acts (preparation)
What stops you?		Protective factors

The level of detail at each stage will depend on the answer to each of these questions. A useful (open) question in this difficult area is: *Can you tell me a bit more about that?*

Note* These thoughts are rarely static, **usually fluctuating**.

○ Thoughts of self-harm (TSH) but no plan.
○ Plans to self-harm—explore what plan is in place and if they have any current (or recent) intention to act on these thoughts.

The best predictor of future behaviour is previous behaviour (see Chapter 15). It is very important to always ask about a history of DSH. If present, using the concepts above, describe (where possible) each episode:

- Method used.
- Whether they took steps to avoid discovery/how they were discovered.
- Degree of planning (left a note, organized affairs, planned the method in detail).
- Treatment needed.
- Their own response to the event.

2.2.3 Past psychiatric history

A **detailed** summary of previous illness. It is not enough to simply say 'past history of depression'. There is a significant difference between 'depression' that is self-limiting, required GP treatment, anti-depressants, or admission to a mental health unit and ECT (electro-convulsive therapy) (see Chapter 17). Equally, assess whether any treatment was effective, what was required, and whether they fully recovered and/or relapsed, required admission (voluntary/involuntary), for how long, etc.

Structured examples include:

- Have they ever had severe depression before?
- Did this require treatment? By whom (GP/psychiatrist)? For how long?
- What did this treatment involve?
  - Psychological.
  - Medication/ECT.
  - Did they recover fully?
  - If they have had multiple episodes of illness:
    - How long in between episodes?
    - Any particular pattern/triggers they can identify?
- Have they ever been admitted (voluntary/involuntary basis—see Chapter 15)? For how long?
- **Note:** Sometimes patients will give a specific name to their diagnosis. It is always important to confirm this with the treating team. Similarly, **always,** check on mental health 'diagnoses' written in the medical notes—they may not necessarily be correct (more detective work).

2.2.4 Past (and current) medical and surgical history

- As in a medical history, details and dates should be given, when available: illnesses/accidents/surgeries and their respective outcomes/treatments.
- 'Systems review', if appropriate.

2.2.5 Family history

Family history and personal history overlap, e.g. details of early childhood, parents, and siblings. In this section, we note any genetic vulnerabilities, and protective (or adverse) events in childhood.

The history should include:

- Parents:
  - Are they still alive? If deceased, when/what age/how?
    - Person's response to the bereavement(s)?
  - Parents' occupation(s).
  - Nature of relationship between parents and patient.

- Siblings:
  - O Patient's position in family relative to other siblings.
  - O Relationship with siblings; deceased siblings.
- Relationships within the family in general.
- Family history of psychiatric illness, suicide.

2.2.6 Personal history

See Practical tips Personal history.

Practical tips Personal history

- At each stage, consider stressors/vulnerability/protective factors.
- Progress in a logical way through the patient's life-stages.
- Consider **what** you are asking and **why** (see the text for examples).

2.2.6.1 Birth and early childhood

Depth of questioning depends on the age of the patient and the presenting complaint:

- Child and adolescent/learning disability psychiatry—parents provide specific details (including developmental milestones).
- Pregnancy/perinatal complications (e.g. pre-term, hypoxia) linked in studies with increased risk for some disorders (e.g. schizophrenia).

Note: A person may disclose a history of childhood sexual abuse. This is a very sensitive topic, and it is usually not appropriate to discuss this—particularly at a first interview or as a student. If, at any stage in the interview, topics arise that you feel are too difficult for you to manage, it is best to politely end the interview, indicating that you will ask a senior member of the team to intervene. Please see guidance and practical tips on how to manage this (and duty of disclosure) in Chapter 1.

2.2.6.2 Education

You are assessing the person's **academic** and **social** functions. Patterns that are evident here are important as they are **predictive** both of **future patterns** and **future vulnerabilities** (see Practical tips—interview questions (education)). Equally, if they are of recent onset, they may indicate an evolving major mental illness or substance abuse.

Key areas are:

- Age at which schooling began and ended (if unusual, why?).
- Move/excluded from school?

- Extra-curricular interests.
- Key areas of function:
  o Ability (academic)—how did they get on at subjects/exams?
  o Social (peers)—how did they get on with peers?
  o Social (authority)—how did they get on with teachers?

Practical tips—interview questions (education)		
Do not assume a specific educational level	Do not stigmatize or judge a particular social style when getting information	
How did you find school-work? Did you do any exams?	How did you get on with other students?	How were your teachers? Did you get on well with them?
Any subjects you particularly liked?	Were you someone who liked to be in the centre of everything, or preferred to keep to yourself?	

You can adapt these questions for subsequent schooling (if appropriate) to ask about second- and third-level education/qualifications.

2.2.6.3 Occupation

The areas are similar to those in education.
For present (and previous) jobs:

- **Ability** to manage the tasks.
- **Social** peers—work colleagues.
- **Social** authority—managers.
- Length of time in each job/reasons for being let go.

2.2.6.4 Relationships

This is a particularly sensitive topic. As always, common sense should be used.

Again, as in previous sections, you are interested in **patterns of behaviour**—whether they have been able to sustain a relationship, and the quality of the relationship.

Note: It is rarely necessary (or appropriate) to take a detailed sexual history in your first interview as a student, unless they are presenting with relevant symptoms and volunteer these. Exceptions would include when taking drug side-effect history, where many of the side-effects may be on sexual function. Again, common sense must prevail in a decision as to how best to proceed with this, particularly for novices/student doctors.

- Number and duration of previous relationships (if any):
  o Any relationship difficulties/abuse?
  o How did the relationship end?

- Current relationship (if any):
  - Duration of relationship?
  - Married/living together?
  - Any relationship difficulties?
  - Partner:
    - Age?
    - Occupation?
    - Health problems (physical or mental health)?
- Children (see Practical tips Children):
  - Names and ages.
  - Health problems (physical or mental health)?
  - Where do they live? Who cares for them mainly?

Practical tips Children

Those dealing with adults who present with mental illness can forget there may be dependant (vulnerable) children. **Always** ask about children.

- Sexual history:
  - Sexual orientation?
  - Age of first sexual experience?
  - Any sexual difficulties?

2.2.7 Substance use, medication, allergies

2.2.7.1 Current medications

A list of <u>all</u> medications, psychotropics (for mental illness), and others:

- Generic names should be used (may include trade names as well).
- Dosage (timings and amount) should also be documented.
- Injected depot medication is especially important (name, dose, frequency, time of last injection).
- Includes herbal or alternative remedies and over the counter (OTC) medications.
- Need to also include items like the oral contraceptive pill (OCP)

2.2.7.2 Allergies

- Precise nature of the allergy (clarify if describing a side-effect or an allergic response).

2.2.7.3 Substance use history

The length of this part of the history will clearly depend on whether or not the person is abusing drugs or alcohol (see Chapter 10).

- Should include licit (e.g. benzodiazepine) and illicit substances:
  - O **Age** at which substance was first used?
  - O **When** was substance last used?
  - O **How often** is the substance used?
  - O **Quantities** of substance used?
  - O Is there evidence of **dependency**/functional **impairment**?
  - O When and for how long (if ever) have they been abstinent?

2.2.8 Forensic history (detail is important)

This provides crucial information about risk of violence (please see Practical tips Interview questions (forensic) and Clinical vignette Forensic assessment in the ED—understanding the perspective of the person you are interviewing).

Practical tips Interview questions (forensic)		
Approach the topic with diplomacy	If there is a history of offences ALWAYS ask for details	
Have you ever had any trouble with the police?* **Some patients will feel the fault lies not with them, but with the law enforcers.*	*What was the charge?* *What exactly happened?* *What age were you?* *Any charges outstanding?** **May influence behaviour.*	*Were you convicted?* *How long were you in prison?** **An indication of the likely seriousness of the offence.*

Clinical vignette Forensic assessment in the ED—understanding the perspective of the person you are interviewing

'It is always important to understand the perspective (and experience) of the person you are assessing, particularly so in a forensic history. This will guide your questions.

'I was taken by my trainee to see a person they had assessed in the ED. As always, I asked the trainee about forensic history or history of violence. The trainee (both capable and enthusiastic) was quite clear that, although the person was recently released from "a spell in prison", this was "only for robbery"—there had been no violence. Closer questioning revealed that the "spell in prison" had been for five years—a lengthy sentence for "only robbery". Explaining to the attendee my surprise that a judge had handed such a lengthy sentence for "robbery", the person admitted "there was an unfortunate complication... the person I was robbing died".

'On another occasion in the ED, the person being assessed, after specific questioning about violence, explained they had had a series of "unfortunate" incidents where they were "obliged" to assault people to "protect themselves" due to the "dangerous" nature of their occupation (disclosed as stealing vehicles to order). This necessitated them carrying a weapon with them at all times to protect themselves from angry owners.' Consultant Liaison Psychiatrist

2.2.9 Current social circumstances

- Where, with whom, do they live?
- Renting or own accommodation?
- Any financial issues (debts, loans, access to benefits, etc.)?
- Overview of their current occupation, current use of substances, and usual leisure activities.
- Can also comment on their available social supports.

2.2.10 Premorbid personality

How would the person have described themselves before they became ill? How would others have described them?

Note When a person is mentally unwell, their account of their premorbid personality may not be an accurate reflection of their true baseline. Some may be overly negative, others overly positive and omit negative aspects, such as a history of aggression.

It is important to look at all aspects of personality—**strengths** as well as **weaknesses**. A good knowledge of personality disorders will help to guide you in this area (see Chapter 5).

2.3 Special circumstances: context and cultural considerations

While psychiatry is a branch of Western medicine, profoundly influenced by Western culture and concepts of disease, many of the core features of mental illness are the same across cultures. However, the content of delusions and hallucinations, and the presentations of stress-related conditions, in particular, are significantly influenced by cultural context. Some conditions are 'culture-bound', i.e. specifically associated with a specific culture (see section 2.3.1). Others, such as anorexia nervosa, originally only described in Western societies, are increasingly seen in other cultural settings, albeit they may focus on physical symptoms (abdominal pain/unable to enjoy food), rather than the more typical symptoms of fear of fatness and altered body image. Questions remain as to the suitability of Western-based classification systems in a non-Western society. **In any assessment, careful consideration of the cultural and societal influences on the manner and form of presentation must be given** (see also Chapter 1).

2.3.1 Examples of cultural context and psychiatric presentation

- Replacement of depressive symptoms with somatic symptoms.
- Abnormal beliefs that may appear delusional in Western context but are culturally appropriate, e.g. beliefs in magic, possession by spirits, demons.
- Apparent disorganization of speech that is actually due to idiosyncrasies in local syntax or difficulty with a language that is not the person's first language.

- Poor engagement or eye contact reflecting historical or cultural distrust of mental health services in the person's country of origin.
- Specific manifestations of distress, termed 'culture-bound syndromes', such as *koro* and *amok*.

2.4 Collateral history (history from relevant others about the patient)

A reliable collateral history is a key part of a psychiatric history. The person's consent is generally required, except in certain circumstances, e.g. where there is a significant risk to the patient or to someone else. Collateral history may be obtained from a family member, a friend, or from other services with which the patient is in contact, e.g. their GP, other mental health services, a school report, if deemed appropriate.

2.5 Summary

Knowledge of the structure and content of history-taking is the first part of clinical assessment. This chapter provides the key structure and questions. The next part of the clinical assessment is the 'examination' of the patient. In mental health you should be doing this (observing and paying close attention to behaviour) **while you are taking the history**. You will then need to probe with specific questions, depending on what you have **heard** in the history and what you have **observed** to date during the interview. These two points will not always coincide (see Chapter 3). The next chapter discusses the specifics of how to 'examine' and how to present these findings in a coherent, structured way (**the mental state examination, MSE**). As always, this will require **knowledge** (of the structure, terms, and underlying illnesses) together with **skill** and **experience**. Practical tips are presented throughout the chapter to help to promote skills. Together, the clinical history and MSE, form the first steps in your clinical assessment.

CHAPTER 3

Mental state examination

CHAPTER FOCUS

What you should know about mental state examination—'what to examine'

- The structure and headings of the MSE.
- Key questions to ask in each section.
- Key observations to make and how to document them.
- Specific examples for:
  - What to ask in sensitive areas.
  - Best terms to use when presenting observations, including official terminology.

3.1 Introduction

The mental state examination (MSE) is the 'physical examination' of psychiatry. It is the examiner's observation of the person's **behaviour and signs** 'here and now'. The history, in contrast, recounts the person's symptoms from time of onset. The two do not always coincide. For example, a person may say they are not hearing voices, but may regularly stop in mid-sentence to look suspiciously at a corner of the room, as if they are responding to voices. Or, a person may say their mood is 'good' but may be sitting in a corner, looking at the floor, weeping silently. Your observations are key. To continue the detective analogy, you are searching for further 'clues' to support what you have found so far in the history. As in a 'physical' examination, specific, precise terms (psychopathology—see Glossary) are used. The MSE is **an account of your observations** of the patient and should **not** take the form of a personal critique (see Practical tips Observations).

Practical tips Observations

- Do not use terms such as 'normal' or 'unusual', as they provide little valid information to others (The word normal may be used to describe speech when there is no disorder evident, e.g. 'speech is normal in rate, tone and volume'.).
- Avoid judgemental terms, e.g. the patient was 'truculent' or 'difficult'. These may indicate deficiencies in the interviewer, rather than the interviewee. Instead describe exactly what was observed, e.g. 'there were significant discrepancies between the history and the observed behaviour' or 'there were discrepancies between the history given and the collateral history'.

3.2 Mental state examination—key headings

The MSE is divided into several headings. Each describes particular aspect of behaviour or illness (psychopathology). **Please refer to the Glossary of psychopathology for terms used in this chapter.** See Figure 3.1 for a useful **mnemonic**.

3.2.1 Appearance and behaviour

Observation is crucial (see Clinical vignette Observation). Observe from the moment you see patients (often before introduction), noting any signs suggestive of illness (or their absence), e.g. social withdrawal (sitting on a bench, eyes downcast, silent) or engagement (speaking on a phone, laughing and smiling).

Clinical vignette Observation

'I learned to start observing even before the interview started, looking through the window before going in. This can yield crucial information. Patients reluctant to confess how badly they were feeling might be lying down, facing the wall, avoiding any social interaction. Others might have given a history of depression and despair, but might be seen laughing, joking, on their mobile phone. These observations were not taken in isolation, but were always important as part of the overall assessment, particularly when there were discrepancies between history and behaviour. I have used these experiences in my own practice as a GP.' GP Trainer

---

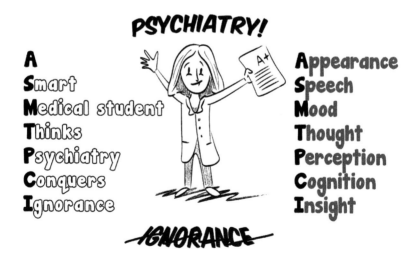

PSYCHIATRY!

A   **A**ppearance
Smart   **S**peech
Medical student **M**ood
Thinks   **T**hought
Psychiatry **P**erception
Conquers **C**ognition
Ignorance **I**nsight

~~IGNORANCE~~

Figure 3.1 A useful mnemonic for mental state examination.
© Eoin Kelleher.

3.2.1.1 Appearance

- General condition/appearance:
  - O Normal weight/underweight/overweight.
  - O Self-care, grooming, dress.
  - O Posture.
- Facial expression—depressed, anxious, mask-like (Parkinsonism).

3.2.1.2 Behaviour

- Seated/relaxed or pacing around/restless.
- Spontaneous, normal, or abnormal movements.
- Eye contact—good, poor, avoidant.
- Social behaviour:
  - O Easy/difficult to establish rapport.
  - O Anxious/distressed (tearful, wringing hands).
  - O Irritable/suspicious/guarded (refuses to sit, keeps distance, or comes too close).
  - O Over-familiar/disinhibited (singing, laughing inappropriately).
  - O Seems to respond to hallucinations (breaking off mid-sentence, staring at a corner of the room, seeming to follow something with his eyes).

3.2.2 Speech

Characteristics of speech (**content** of speech reflects **thoughts**):

- Rate, volume, tone (variation in the pitch of the voice) (e.g. speaks loudly, rapidly, impossible to interrupt—suggestive of mania).
- Quantity.
- Spontaneity (markedly reduced, e.g. depression).
- Fluency—difficulties with the production of speech (may reflect local problems—dysarthria, or more complex, central issues, e.g. dysphasia or abnormalities of thought processes discussed below).

If there are abnormalities, document examples.

3.2.3 Mood and affect

Mood (emotional state over a prolonged time) may be depressed (low), elated (high), or normal (euthymic/normothymic), congruent/incongruent. If not already asked in the presenting complaint, ask here about (and document) aspects such as diurnal mood variation, insomnia, early morning wakening.

Affect (emotional state at a particular moment in time) is also included under this heading:

- Reactive (to the interviewer).
- Restricted/flat (reduced).

- Blunted (lacks emotional response).
- Labile (fluctuates rapidly).

3.2.4 Thought

3.2.4.1 Thought form

Abnormalities in the form (i.e. structure) of thought. Examples include circumstantiality, flight of ideas, loosening of associations, 'thought blocking' (see the Glossary for definitions).

3.2.4.2 Thought content

The contents/subjects of thoughts are usually closely connected to mental state, e.g. themes of worthlessness or hopelessness (depression), grandiosity (mania), persecution (psychosis). If these are held with delusional intensity, they will be described as persecutory/grandiose delusions, etc. Recurrent, intrusive thoughts, images, or impulses (seen with obsessive–compulsive disorder (OCD)) will also be documented here, and any associated compulsions (see the Glossary for definitions and Clinical vignette Example of abnormalities of thought form and content (mania)).

> **Clinical vignette** Example of abnormalities of thought form and content (mania)
>
> 'In addition to marked pressure of speech, Mr X exhibited marked flight of ideas, switching rapidly from one thought to the next. A connection between topics was evident, though at times this was unusual, e.g. through clang [see Glossary] associations "Dr Dunne, you are done now". There were prominent grandiose delusions (convinced he had supernatural powers).' Example of abnormalities of thought form and content reported by psychiatrist (mania)

Thoughts about self-harm (or, if relevant, harm to others) should be enquired about here, if not previously addressed in the presenting complaint (see Chapter 2).

3.2.5 Perception

Abnormalities of perception (illusions or hallucinations) and their type (auditory, visual, olfactory, gustatory, tactile) are noted here (see Practical tips Hallucinations). You must know what these terms mean and differences between, for example, illusions and hallucinations (see the Glossary for definitions).

If **auditory hallucinations** are present, you will need to describe them in detail (second or third person), as this can have diagnostic significance:

- 2nd person: voices speaking to the patient includes 'command hallucinations' (giving orders, e.g. *kill yourself, you are worthless*) (associated with **risk** of acting on them).

- 3rd person: speaking about the patient (discussing him or providing a running commentary on his actions, e.g. *he is putting on his shoes, he is tying his laces*, the latter particularly associated with schizophrenia—Schneiderian first rank symptom) (see Chapter 7).

Visual hallucinations (e.g. seeing spiders running up the wall or rats on the floor) are typically associated with physical/organic illness, e.g. delirium tremens.

Practical tips Hallucinations

- **Visual** hallucinations suggest **organic**/physical illness.
- **Auditory** hallucinations suggest primary **mental** illness.

3.2.6 Cognitive function/memory
This section provides a brief overview. Please see Chapter 11 for more detailed examples.

- Note the person's **concentration** and **attention** during the interview and their understanding of the interview process. More formal testing includes:
  - O Orientation to time, place, and person.
  - O Spell WORLD forwards and then backwards.
  - O Months of the year backwards.
  - O Serial 7s or digit span (subtract 7 from 100 and continue to take 7 from the answer or remember a series of numbers).
- Comment also on a person's general language ability from the history and mental state:
  - O Fluency, rate, and spontaneity of speech (can indicate dysarthria or dysphasia).
  - O Grammatical errors, paraphasia (use of unintended syllables).
  - O Difficulty in naming objects (nominal dysphasia).
  - O Difficulty in comprehension (further defined by giving two and three-stage commands) (receptive dysphasia).
- If there are concerns about the person's cognitive function, this can be tested more formally by neuro-psychologists.

3.2.7 Insight
This refers to the person's understanding of their symptoms.
  Insight has several levels of belief:

- There is something wrong.
- This is due to illness.
- The illness is mental (or physical).

- There is a treatment available.
- The treatment will help them.
- They will accept the treatment.

Insight is not an all-or-nothing phenomenon—the person's level of insight will determine whether they will engage with treatment.

3.3 Summary

Conducting a proper MSE requires knowledge of an appropriate structure, and key questions, outlined in this chapter. Carefully document your observations, with specific examples, where appropriate. The MSE, and the history, are the first steps to clinical assessment. These are then summarized and considered in the formulation (see Chapter 4), to provide structure in order to:

- Understand why the patient has presented (why now, why this patient, why this illness).
- Guide investigations.
- Propose an appropriate intervention.

Proposing a diagnosis: classifications, formulation, and investigations

> **CHAPTER FOCUS**
>
> What you should know about proposing a diagnosis and initial management
> - Suggest possible diagnoses and understand current diagnostic classifications.
> - Construct a formulation—why this person, in this way, at this time?
> - Generate a bio-psycho-social model of understanding and management.
> - Propose appropriate investigations.

4.1 Introduction

Previous chapters have explained how to set up, and conduct, the clinical assessment. This chapter elaborates on:

- How to use this information to generate an initial, 'working' diagnosis (the likely nature of the underlying illness)—**diagnostic classification systems**.
- An understanding of why the person may have presented in this manner— **a formulation**.
- Appropriate **investigations** to support (or refute) this working hypothesis.

As diagnosis in mental health still relies almost exclusively on clinical expertise in history-taking and examination, it is crucial to constantly consider and review the working diagnosis. This is particularly important when the person first presents, as once a diagnosis is 'established' it can persist in the medical notes as 'irrefutable fact', particularly when patients with mental ill-health present in medical settings where there is less familiarity with diagnostic systems (see Clinical vignette Diagnostic systems). Continuing the analogy from Chapter 2, you must still be in 'detective' mode, constantly reviewing and re-analysing the evidence to support or refute your diagnosis (Figure 4.1).

> **Clinical vignette** Diagnostic systems
>
> 'I confess to having been bewildered by psychiatry terms. They all seemed the same—"EUPD", "BAD", "BPD"—yet I knew they often had serious implications for optimizing patient care in a medical setting where I worked (and where they often presented). I realized I would have to learn about, and understand, how mental health diagnoses were made and what they meant.' Medical Registrar

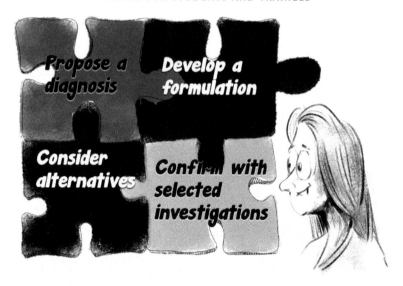

Figure 4.1 Proposing a diagnosis—continue to be a detective.
© Eoin Kelleher.

4.2 Diagnostic classification systems

Classification systems in mental disorders act as guides to promote reliable diagnoses. There are two internationally recognized diagnostic classification systems:

- ICD-10: International Classification of Diseases (the number '10' refers to the edition in current clinical use; version 11 is currently being introduced).
- DSM-5: Diagnostic and Statistical Manual of Mental Disorders (the number '5' refers to the edition in current clinical use).

Diagnostic classification systems seek to facilitate:

- **Clinical care** by promoting:
  - ○ Clarity of diagnosis.
  - ○ Clear communication between clinicians.
  - ○ Accountability, especially for involuntary care.
- **Education:**
  - ○ Patients to understand their experiences.
  - ○ Families and the public to understand mental illness.
- **Research:**
  - ○ Identification of subgroups selected for research interventions.
  - ○ Assessment of research studies.

- Service planning:
  - Based on research outcomes.
  - Based on public health research.

However, there are many **criticisms** of diagnostic classifications. These include the arguments that they may:

- Be too restrictive, reducing a person to a single item.
- Fail to capture the richness of any one presentation.
- Fail to recognize the overlap between several conditions.
- Cause the clinician to miss other salient features.
- Become 'pejorative labels'.
- Cause the medicalization of non-health behaviours.

While knowledge of the diagnostic criteria for any condition is important, transferring this into the clinical expertise to recognize, quantify, and designate these complex presentations and to distinguish them from normal variations and/ or responses to stress, requires considerable clinical training and experience. Furthermore, it must always be recognized that a diagnosis of mental illness will be heavily influenced by a range of factors within the individual, which include personality, age, cognitive function, the presence (or absence) of co-morbid medical illness, and the presence (or absence) of social support and stressors. Both ICD and DSM emphasize this broad approach and warn against 'tick-box' diagnosis (see Table 4.1).

Some of the criticisms levelled at the categorical nature of classification were eased, a little, by multi-axial diagnostic systems. In DSM IV, this meant that any presentation was considered over five axes:

Axis 1: major mental illness.
Axis 2: personality and intellectual disability.
Axis 3: medical diagnoses.
Axis 4: psychosocial impairment.
Axis 5: global assessment of function.

Table 4.1 Practical tips Remember advantages and disadvantages of diagnoses

Advantages—can provide	Disadvantages—can be
Clarity of diagnosis	Restrictive
Clear communication	Perjorative
Accountability	Medicalize
Education	
Structure for planning and research	

DSM-5 has removed these axes, subsuming Axes 1, 2, and 3, and suggesting separate notations for those features on Axes 4 and 5. For clinicians, particularly students in training, the concept of the multi-axial system is helpful in ensuring that the wider context of a person's presentation is considered, and while it may no longer be part of DSM-5, it is a useful clinical strategy.

ICD-10 also suggests a multi-axial system, but these are very broad (and probably less useful for the student).

Main features of DSM-5 and ICD-10
DSM-5 (published 2014):

- American-based, published by the American Psychiatric Association.
- Provides a coherent, focused, point-based descriptive account of disorders and their impact.
- Only available in English.
- Manual must be purchased.

ICD-10 (published 1990, ICD 11 implementation due 2021/22):

- European-based, published by the World Health Organization (WHO).
- Largely a narrative account.
- Available in multiple languages.
- Freely available on the internet.
- Classifies all diseases (see Chapter 5).

There are differences between the two systems with respect to both the disorders included and the diagnostic criteria. ICD is generally used within a European context. Students will **not** be expected to know individual codes but will need to have a broad understanding of diagnostic categories and be aware of the main diagnostic criteria for the major disorders.

4.3 Proposing a diagnosis

After the first interview with the patient, you should have several potential diagnoses in mind. The process builds on your interview and mental state examination. You should continue to 'be a detective' (Figure 4.1).

- The most likely diagnosis should be written first. Subsequent diagnoses are listed in order of decreasing likelihood.
- You need to be able to justify your proposed diagnosis using 'evidence' from your history and MSE.
- A person's **diagnosis may change over time**, as new information becomes available or as clinical features become more apparent.
- A person may meet criteria for more than one diagnosis. **All** potential diagnoses should be documented.

- The proper diagnostic terms should be used. For example, simply documenting 'depression' gives little information as to the severity of their illness. Documenting 'severe depressive episode with psychotic symptoms' is much more useful. Management plans are developed on the basis of symptom severity, amongst other factors. In the same way that angina is managed differently from a myocardial infarct (MI) (even though the underlying pathology may be similar), a mild depressive episode is approached very differently to a severe depressive episode with psychosis
- Diagnosis should also include a preliminary assessment of the patient's personality (see Chapter 5).
- The patient's overall level of functioning should be noted (see discussion on multi-axial classification above).
- A person may not meet criteria for any mental illness and it is also important to document the <u>absence</u> of a psychiatric disorder.
- Always consider a physical cause. This must be excluded first, as management will be very different.

4.4 Formulation (as distinct from diagnosis or summary)

The **summary** is an impartial, objective description of the patient's presentation. The **diagnosis** describes a patient's presentation within a framework that identifies similarities between them and others with similar presentations (e.g. major depressive episode). The **formulation** is the clinician's synthesis of all the facts about the patient to create a management plan for this **individual** (see Practical tips Formulation).

Practical tips Formulation

- Diagnosis describes how patients are similar.
- Formulation describes how each patient is distinct.

The **formulation** of a patient is based on an extensive history and an accurate mental state examination. It helps us to understand:

- **Why** this person became ill.
- **Why** this illness.
- **Why** now.

Typically, one starts with a summary of the case, then examines contributing factors. These factors are usually divided into groups:

- **Predisposing factors**: what made this person vulnerable to developing the illness?
- **Precipitating factors**: what was the trigger for the illness?

Table 4.2 Example of a bio-psycho-social approach to formulation

	Biological	Psychological	Social
Predisposing	Family history of mental illness.	Early life adversity (childhood trauma or abuse). Maladaptive coping strategies.	Growing up in a socially-fragmented environment.
Precipitating	Non-adherence to prescribed medication.	Breakdown of marital relationship. Redundancy from work.	Financial difficulties. Living in homeless accommodation.
Perpetuating	Continued non-adherence to medication. Co-morbid alcohol use.	Criticism from estranged partner.	Inappropriate accommodation.
Protective	Healthy diet and life-style.	Good support from family of origin.	Community involvement and connection.

- **Perpetuating factors**: what is maintaining the illness?
- **Protective factors**, promoting resilience, should also be considered.

The above factors can then be further divided into biological, psychological and social factors, a bio-psycho-social approach (see Table 4.2). In practice, there is often overlap between psychological and social factors.

4.5 Investigations

Mental health clinicians rely largely on their clinical skills to make a diagnosis. This is supported by appropriate investigations.

4.5.1 Collateral history

The most important initial investigation is **collateral history** from relatives, close friends, and previous medical care, particularly from GPs. **No assessment is complete without a collateral history.**

4.5.2 Baseline physical health and investigations

Physical health must **always** be considered. Physical examination (and investigations) can:

1. Ensure a medical disorder is not the underlying cause.
2. Identify physical sequelae of psychiatric disorders.

3. Identify adverse effects of prescribed medications.
4. Establish baseline physical parameters, e.g. body mass index, waist circumference, electrocardiogram (ECG), etc.

When ordering an investigation, it is important to think about **why** you are doing this test and how the information yielded will change your management plan (see also Chapter 17).

4.5.3 Blood tests

- Full blood count (FBC):
  - O Low haemoglobin causes fatigue (may be mistaken for a symptom of depression).
  - O Alcohol abuse may lead to raised mean corpuscular volume (MCV).
  - O The antipsychotic, Clozapine, can cause neutropaenia. Baseline FBC is, therefore, required before, and monitored during, treatment.
- Liver enzymes, liver function tests (LFTs):
  - O A person who is drinking to excess may have deranged LFTs—a raised gamma-glutamyl transferase (GGT) may be an early warning sign of liver dysfunction in alcohol abuse (or may be secondary to medication).
- B12/folate:
  - O In older people, B12 deficiency is one of the reversible causes of dementia.
- Thyroid function tests (TFTs):
  - O Hyperthyroidism is associated with symptoms that can mimic anxiety.
  - O Hypothyroidism is associated with symptoms that mimic depression.
  - O Monitored in lithium therapy due to effects of lithium on the thyroid.
- Renal function tests (RFTs or UEC—urea, electrolytes and creatinine):
  - O The mood stabilizer lithium is renally excreted and long-term lithium use is associated with nephropathy. Renal impairment (and age) may affect dosing schedule (see Chapters 6 and 17).
- Prolactin:
  - O Antipsychotics may cause an increase in prolactin due to their effect on dopamine level (particularly risperidone). Increasingly, routine monitoring is now requested.
- Metabolic parameters (lipids and glucose):
  - O The newer antipsychotics are particularly associated with 'metabolic syndrome' (see Chapter 7)

4.6 Electrocardiogram (ECG)

- The antipsychotics and some of the antidepressants can affect the ECG to varying degrees (prolonging a specific measurement on the ECG called the (corrected) QT interval (QTc)).
- Baseline ECG can identify any pre-existing pathology, and follow-up ECGs are used if symptomatic or in a high-risk category.

4.7 Computerized tomography (CT)/magnetic resonance imaging (MRI) of the brain

These are not routinely carried out but may be justified on the basis of the presentation, for example:

- First presentation of a psychotic illness.
- Symptoms suggestive of an underlying neurological disorder.
- Atypical symptoms.
- Not responding to treatment as expected,

4.8 Other assessment tools and the multi-disciplinary team (MDT)

Assessments from other members of the multi-disciplinary team, such as clinical psychology, social workers, mental health nurses, and occupational therapists, are key in assessment and management (see Chapter 16). There are a variety of assessment tools (questionnaires and scales) that can help in diagnosis and/or help to monitor response to treatment. They are also used in research settings. These assessment scales can be self-rated or observer-rated, and vary in complexity and validity. Training is required before one can administer certain rating scales. They must **always** be interpreted with care, in a clinical context. Unquestioning acceptance of the results of a psychological test in isolation can be very unhelpful. More complex scales will require the expertise of a clinical psychologist, key members of any team delivering clinical care, or the speciality responsible for the assessment (e.g. occupational therapist (OT)).

As a student, you should know the CAGE questionnaire, an easy tool to help identify alcohol dependence (see Chapter 10). You should be aware of some of the other scales, as they will be discussed in team meetings; however, you will not need to know them in detail (examples below). Specific assessment tools relating to assessment of memory or those used in subspecialties, such as child and adolescent psychiatry or forensic psychiatry, are discussed in the relevant chapters.

4.9 Examples of assessment tools (questionnaires and scales)

4.9.1 General Items

4.9.1.1 General health questionnaire (GHQ)

- Self-rated.
- Screening tool for psychiatric illness designed to be used in primary care or general medical settings.

4.9.1.2 Global assessment of functioning (GAF)

- Clinician rated.
- 100 items.
- Looks at overall level of functioning (psychological, social, occupation).

4.9.1.3 Clinical global impression (CGI)

- Two items:
  - ○ Global severity—clinician rates the severity of illness relative to others with the same diagnosis.
  - ○ Global change—rates change relative to a baseline assessment.
- Can be patient- or carer-rated.

4.9.1.4 Structured clinical interview for DSM (SCID)

- DSM is the American classification system for psychiatric disorders; it is now in its 5th edition (DSM-5).
- The SCID is a clinician-administered assessment that takes the form of a semi-structured clinical interview.
- It can be used as a part of the normal assessment of a patient but, in practice, it is usually used in research/epidemiological studies.
- There is a version, the SCID II, which is used in personality disorders.

4.9.5 Mood disorders

4.9.5.1 Beck depression inventory (BD®-II)

- Self-rated.
- 21 statements: four possible responses for each.
- Assesses the patient's symptoms over the preceding week.
- A score of >17 indicates moderate depression; >30 indicates a more severe depressive illness

4.9.5.2 Hospital anxiety and depression scale (HADS)

HADS is particularly useful in a hospital setting, as it is less reliant on 'biological' symptoms:

- Self-rated.
- 14 items.
- Gives scores for anxiety component and for depressive component.

4.9.5.3 Edinburgh post-natal depression scale

- Self-rated.
- Ten questions; four possible responses for each.

- Typically used at weeks 6–8 post-partum.
- Assesses the patient's symptoms over the preceding week.
- Gives suggestions for referral/management based on score.

4.9.6 Obsessive–compulsive disorder

4.9.6.1 Yale-Brown obsessive–compulsive scale (YBOCS)

- Self-rated and clinician versions available.
- Ten items relating to obsessions and compulsions.
- Five-point Likert scale.

4.9.7 Psychotic disorders

4.9.7.1 Brief psychiatric rating scale (BPRS)

- Clinician-rated.
- Primary use is in schizophrenia.
- Measures psychotic and non-psychotic symptoms.

4.9.7.2 Positive and negative symptoms of schizophrenia (PANSS)

- Clinician-rated.
- Used to assess severity of symptoms.
- Also used to monitor change in presentation/response to treatment.

4.9.7.3 Abnormal involuntary movement scale (AIMS)

- Clinician-rated.
- 12 items rated 0–4.
- Used to assess for side-effects of antipsychotic medication.

4.9.8 Substance use disorders
CAGE Questionnaire (see Chapter 10).

4.9.9 Psychopathy/psychopathic personality disorder
The **PCL-R (psychopathy checklist-revised)** is used as part of an assessment of suspected psychopathy and is usually carried out in a forensic setting. The assessment includes a thorough review of past history and relevant records, as well as a number of clinical interviews. **Use of this tool requires specific training and experience.**

4.10 Summary
Organizing information collected in the history and MSE to generate a working diagnosis is the first step to therapeutic intervention. Constructing a formulation,

using a bio-psycho-social model, with the help of the MDT, helps to understand the presentation in **this particular person**. Ancillary investigations help to both support a diagnosis and guide appropriate management. A further factor to consider is the person's **personality**—every illness presents in the context of the person's personality, which will shape and influence how they present. The next chapter discusses personality disorders and how to assess them. Subsequent chapters give information on common and specialist clinical conditions, which you will use in your detective role to customize your history-taking and MSE as you seek evidence to support or refute your working diagnosis. Good luck!

Personality disorders

5.1 Introduction

Every presentation occurs in a person with a pre-existing, 'pre-morbid', personality. This personality will have a profound impact on presentation and interventions.

5.2 Personality—definition

The term 'personality' refers to enduring patterns of behaviour, deeply ingrained attitudes, and responses, typically present from adolescence, persisting throughout adult life, and manifesting across different situations. It defines our interests, how we interact with others, and how we respond to stress. Personality is likely to be contributed to by both genetic and environmental factors. Studies on children's temperament suggest that the foundations of personality are evident from an early age.

5.2.1 Personality—a warning

There are those who argue we should not use the term personality/personality disorder, that it is used only as a means of 'labelling'. It is important **not to use the term as a pejorative label**. It will only be pejorative if you use it in that manner. Consideration of underlying ingrained patterns of behaviour is an important contribution to understanding a person's presentation. Some people will not have any underlying major mental illness, but will repeatedly present with distress and difficulty in managing. Often the underlying difficulty is their patterns of behaviour, deeply ingrained and persistent, present since adolescence, and causing them significant distress and harm, i.e. their personality. Recognizing these patterns is the first step to providing an intervention. Finally, those with personality disorders are at increased risk of developing a mental illness.

5.3 Personality disorder—the concept

Personality exists on a spectrum. Everyone has traits that can be strengths or weaknesses. A person is said to have a personality disorder if aspects of their personality cause significant distress or difficulty for them and/or those around them. There is usually marked functional impairment, difficulties with interpersonal relationships and emotional responses. These difficulties are persistent and pervasive, and are not due to illness, although unhelpful personality traits can certainly be exacerbated by co-morbid mental or physical illness or stress. Personality disorders are generally not diagnosed before the age of 18 years, as personality is quite changeable up until our 20s. Personality disorder is only diagnosed when the person, or others, suffers because of these traits (see Practical tips Personality disorder diagnosis).

5.4 Personality disorders—the categories

While consideration of patterns of ingrained behaviour (personality traits) helps to understand clinical presentations, the category of personality disorder is a confusing one. Many of the 'categories' are artificial. Furthermore, there are several differences in the categories between ICD-10 and DSM-5, adding to the confusion. (see Table 5.1 for comparisons). People often exhibit traits of several disorders. The same limitations discussed in the chapter on diagnostic classification systems apply here. Often, however, **an overall pattern** of behaviour fits with one main category.

Table 5.1 Comparison of personality disorders ICD-10, DSM-5

ICD-10	DSM-5
Paranoid	Paranoid
Schizoid	Schizoid
Categorized under schizophrenia in ICD 10	Schizotypal
Dissocial	Antisocial
Emotionally unstable, impulsive type Emotionally unstable, borderline type	Borderline
Histrionic	Histrionic
	Narcissistic
Anxious/avoidant	Avoidant
Anankastic	Obsessive–compulsive
Dependent	Dependent

Finally, it is important to note that many patients will either not have a full-blown personality disorder, or you cannot properly assess it (particularly after one assessment). It is usually possible, however, to note a person's personality traits.

When these traits are then presented in the context of a multi-axial system, it provides both a useful overview of the clinical presentation, and helps to guide any psychological intervention (see Clinical vignette Traits).

Clinical vignette Traits

'Mrs X is a 55-year-old widow who presents with mixed anxiety and depressive symptoms in the context of pre-morbid obsessional personality traits (a drive for perfection and heightened sensitivity to criticism) and a recent diagnosis of stage 2 breast cancer.' Psychiatrist

5.5 Personality disorders–demographics

- Prevalence in the community is about 10%.
- In primary care settings, for about 7% of those attending for mental health reasons, the core difficulty is personality disorder (PD).
- In psychiatric outpatients, about 40% of patients will have a personality disorder (this is the primary diagnosis in 5–15%).
- For psychiatric inpatients, the prevalence rate is higher (about 50%).
- Up to 75% of prisoners meet criteria for a personality disorder (dissocial PD is the most common).

Practical tips Personality disorder diagnosis

Personality disorder is only diagnosed when the person, or others, suffers because of the traits.

5.6 Specific personality disorders (ICD-10 criteria)

Students will not be expected to know all the details of each type but should be aware of the different categories and key features of the more common presentations. Rather than long, detailed discussions about each potential personality disorder, the disorders are presented in the form of tables, with lists of their most distinctive traits, accompanied by a mnemonic to help you remember them. This will allow you, if you come across a particular trait, to search for other traits usually associated with it (continuing the theme of a detective searching for clues to support or refute your working diagnosis). The personality types are presented in a particular order (see Tables 5.2–5.9). Those that are most helpful as concepts

Table 5.2 Anankastic (obsessional) personality disorder

Anankastic (obsessional) PD key traits	Mnemonic	'Helpful' obsessional personality traits
Indecisive, afraid of making mistake	I	As with most personality 'disorders', some of these traits, when present to a lesser degree, may be helpful, e.g. an individual may be reliable, organized, determined, precise, keen to do well, sensitive to feedback.
Perfectionistic, so preoccupied by minor details is unable to function	P	
Unable to adapt to change, needs routine, inflexible	A	
Sensitive to criticism (concerned will be judged badly)	S	
Meanness with money due to preoccupation with using it incorrectly, becoming penniless	M	
Unexpressed anger, particularly when others interfere with their routines	U	
Guilt—exaggerated sense of morality, preoccupation with doing the right thing	G	

Table 5.3 Dissocial personality disorder

Dissocial (anti-social) PD* key traits	Mnemonic	'Helpful' dissocial personality traits
Guilt or remorse (lack of), dismissive of social norms/obligations	G	It is more difficult to consider dissocial personality traits as in any way constructive. In popular literature, there are those who argue that some of these traits, in milder form, may confer advantage in competitive business settings.
Impulsive, with a low threshold for frustration and aggression, substance abuse, criminal record	I	
Relationships (lack of), callous, lack of empathy	R	
Learn (failure to learn) from mistakes, blame others for their own behaviour	L	
Superficially charming (may be) but can't maintain loving relationships (often characterized by cruelty), unstable work record	S	

Note: *Psychopathic PD is probably best conceptualized as a severe form of dissocial personality disorder. These individuals are considered at high risk of violence (see Chapter 15). There is often a history of conduct disorder in childhood.

Table 5.4 Paranoid personality disorder

Paranoid PD key traits	Mnemonic	'Helpful' paranoid personality traits
Suspicious and distrustful of others (to extreme degree)	S	It is difficult to conceptualize paranoid personality traits as helpful, except, perhaps, that people with these traits are likely to be very careful in their interactions with others and run less risk of engaging in unhelpful situations or relationships.
Sensitive (to extreme degree), easily takes offence to perceived slights/insults	S	
Self-important, excessive sense of personal rights, can be litigious (believes others have tricked him)	S	

clinically (either most frequently encountered or easiest to conceptualize, particularly for students), are presented first. The disorders listed later are less commonly used (and probably less helpful) concepts in clinical settings today. In each case, the main traits/behaviours associated with the disorder are listed, together with a mnemonic to aid memory.

5.6.1 Note: 'helpful' personality traits

Examples of where particular traits might be 'helpful' (to remind the reader that everyone has patterns of behaviour that vary in their helpfulness) are also included (Figure 5.1). Thus, for example, one might be quite happy if one's surgeon had some obsessional personality traits (attention to detail, striving for perfection, following a routine prior to every operation). It is only when these traits become extreme, leading to distress or harm to the person or others, that they suggest disorder. In the example given, for example, this might be a surgeon so dedicated to perfection that they hesitate before every decision, unable to proceed during an operation in case they make the wrong choice.

Table 5.5 Schizoid personality disorder

Schizoid personality disorder key traits	Mnemonic	'Helpful' schizoid personality traits
Aloof/cold, reduced capacity for emotion or affection	A	Some of these traits, when present to a lesser degree, may be beneficial. An individual can be rational, detached, and unemotional in making difficult decisions in organizations, for example.
Solitary, prefer their own company	Solitary	
Introverted and introspective	Individual	

Table 5.6 Emotionally unstable personality disorder (EUPD)

Emotionally unstable PD (impulsive type) key traits	Mnemonic	'Helpful' EUPD personality traits
Emotional dysregulation, difficulty controlling emotional responses, 'moods' vary rapidly* (extreme in borderline PD see 'Emotionally unstable PD (borderline type)' in this table)	Every	Patients with EUPD are so often overwhelmed by their emotions and their responses, it is difficult to conceptualize of instances when this can be helpful. Marsha Linehan, however, who describes herself as having had borderline personality disorder, studied psychology and used her knowledge to develop dialectical behaviour therapy (DBT) a therapy used in EUPD.
Outbursts of emotion (particularly anger)	Other	
Unpredictable in behaviour/ reactions	University	
Emotionally unstable PD (borderline type) Above features with:		
Sensitive (extremely) to rejection (real or perceived)	Student	
Uncertainty re sense of self, life-goals, sexuality	Unfairly	
Relationships intense and unstable	Receives	
Emptiness, often described as chronic passive death wish	Exceptional	
Maladaptive coping mechanisms prominent (self-harm, substance abuse), often in response to rejection, used as means to avoid being abandoned	Marks	

*Marked difficulty regulating emotions (usual term is **affective instability**):

• Emotions (often described by the person as 'moods') seem to vary greatly and can change within the space of minutes/hours.

• The person generally has little sense of control over these 'mood swings'.

Of all the terms used in an unhelpful way, EUPD is, perhaps, the one most commonly misused. Terms such as 'attention-seeking', referring to acts of self-harm, are very unhelpful concepts. These behaviours are best understood as maladaptive strategies used to cope with intense and overwhelming emotions and/or as a means of expressing distress and/or eliciting care from others.

Table 5.7 Histrionic personality disorder

Histrionic PD key traits	Mnemonic	'Helpful' histrionic traits
Dramatic in manner	Dramatic	When present to a lesser degree, such traits may be considered interesting and engaging.
Centre of attention (need to be) with little consideration for the feelings of others	Chemistry	
Shallow, fleeting emotions	Students	
Self-deception, seem to believe in stories, even when clearly not true	Seemingly	
Exaggerated displays of anger/distress/joy, which pass quickly	Enjoy	
Novelty and excitement needed, easily bored	Novel	
Superficial relationships, flirtatious and affectionate but with limited capacity for a deeper emotional connection	Structures	

Table 5.8 Anxious personality disorder

Anxious/avoidant PD key traits	Mnemonic	'Helpful' anxious personality traits
Anxious and apprehensive	A	Possibly may help to ensure makes 'safe' decisions, but generally these traits not very helpful.
Fear scrutiny from others	Stitch	
Insecure and excessively cautious, particularly of new people/situations	In	
Timid, avoid responsibility, exaggerate risks	Time	
Limited social circle but seek relationships with others (in contrast to schizoid PD)	Saves	

Table 5.9 Dependent personality disorder

Dependent PD key traits	Mnemonic	'Helpful' dependent personality traits
Relies on others to make all decisions for them	Regular	Perhaps, in minor forms, may promote working as part of a team.
Subjugate their own needs, passively comply with others	Study	
See themselves as being unable to cope with day to day life	Can	
Excessive need to be cared for/minded	Cause	
Fear of abandonment	Abandonment	

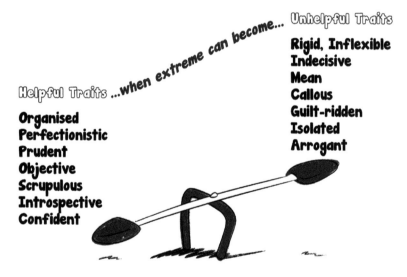

Figure 5.1 The balancing act of personality traits.
© Eoin Kelleher.

The concepts of 'helpful' personality traits can also be useful to engage psycho-therapeutically with patients, as it acknowledges that personality traits:

- Are an inherent, long-lasting part of someone's behaviour and make-up.
- Have often been used successfully by that person in many areas of their life up to now.
- Will require significant work to adapt and change them, if change is needed.

This helps to view any discussion on personality as a useful one, reducing the risk of 'pejorative labelling' referred to above.

5.7 Treatment

Given that personality disorders are, by definition, life-long, enduring, and per-vasive, effecting change can be very difficult, if not impossible. Psychotherapy is generally the mainstay of treatment. Cognitive behaviour therapy (focusing on coping strategies and core beliefs), dialectical behaviour therapy (EUPD-bor-derline) and mentalization-based therapy (EUPD-borderline) may be helpful (see Chapter 16).

5.8 Summary

Personality refers to deeply ingrained, pervasive patterns of behaviour (traits) that influence how people present. When these traits are extreme or unhelpful and present in a constellation of patterns, they may suggest a specific person-ality disorder. However, minor or individual traits can be helpful to the individual. Furthermore, it is important to recognize that, at the very least, people have usually used this coping strategy for a very long time. It is important, therefore, to assess coping styles and strategies; to acknowledge these will have both helpful and unhelpful consequences, and to use these to influence intervention and out-come. Usually, personality is seen within the context of another disorder, such as depression or OCD. Some, particularly psychopathy and borderline personality disorder, present frequently in particular settings (e.g. forensic, emergency).

CHAPTER 6

Mood disorders

What you should know about mood disorders
- How to **recognize** depression and mania.
- How to initially **treat** both.
- Be aware that both can exist **with,** and/or be caused by, a **medical condition/** treatment.
- Recognize that mood disorders can **adversely** affect patients' **function** and physical illness, if present.

6.1 Introduction

Mood disorders are so-called because the core feature is an **abnormality of mood** that is *persistent* and *pervasive*. The term **mood** refers to a sustained emotional state that defines the person's experience. There are two major disorders of mood: depressive disorder (also termed unipolar depression) and bipolar affective disorder. The key difference between the two is the occurrence of both elevated (mania) and depressed mood in bipolar disorder. Two other mood disorders, cyclothymia and dysthymia, will also be discussed. Mildly elevated mood is called hypomania.

The **terminology** of mood disorders can be confusing, both within ICD and because of differences between ICD and DSM (see Chapter 4). Table 6.1 provides a simplified version of the main categories.

6.2 Depressive disorder

Brief feelings of sadness or anger in response to challenges are part of normal life experience. The clinical term 'depression' should be reserved for those with a **pervasive** change of mood, i.e. deterioration in mood that **persists across** different situations, that **endures** for a prolonged time with **little or no variability**, and with **distinctive patterns** of associated symptoms (see Clinical vignette Severe depressive episode).

6.2.1 Core features of depression

- **Pervasive low mood**: minimal variation in mood over the day; worst on wakening in the morning, improving as the day progresses, known as **diurnal mood variation (DMV)** (associated with moderate/severe depression).
- **Reduced capacity for pleasure (anhedonia**—total inability to feel pleasure/ enjoyment).

Table 6.1 Simplified representation of categories for mood disorder episodes*

Select mood presentation	Select pattern of episode presentation		Select severity of current episode	Identify if psychotic features (current episode)
Depressed OR	Single	Single episode	Mild	With
		Manic episode		
		OR		Without
		Depressive episode	Moderate	
	OR	Recurrent episodes		
		Recurrent depressive disorder *(depressive episodes only)*		
		OR	Severe	
Elevated	Recurrent (≥ two episodes)	Bipolar affective disorder *(manic+/– depressive episodes)*		
Elevated or depressed (mild) **not** fulfilling criteria for episodes	Persistent	Dysthymia *mood low* Cyclothymia *mood low and (mildly) high, cycles*	N/A	N/A

* **Example:** 'Recurrent depressive disorder, current episode depressed, moderately severe, without psychotic symptoms'.

Source: Data from World Health Organization. (2004) . *ICD-10: international statistical classification of diseases and related health problems: tenth revision*, 2nd edn.

- Sleep disturbance (insomnia):
  - ○ **Initial insomnia:** difficulty initiating sleep.
  - ○ **Middle insomnia:** difficulty maintaining sleep (wakening throughout the night).
  - ○ **Early morning wakening:** found in moderate/severe depression, typically wakes at least 2 h before their usual waking time, unable to resume sleep, and feels ill-at-ease or distressed. Often associated with DMV.
  - ○ People may report a mix of the above sleep difficulties.

- ○ Some people may report sleeping excessively but their sleep is not refreshing (atypical).
- **Anorexia** (appetite loss)—there may be associated **weight loss**.
- **Anergia** fatigue or lack of energy (some patients may present as fidgety, restless but still report feeling lethargic).
- Reduced, or no, **motivation**.
- Poor **concentration** (often associated with memory difficulties).
- Reduced **libido** (under-reported).
- Feelings and thoughts of **worthlessness** or excessive **guilt**:
  - ○ Ruminate on past events and perceived failings or mistakes.
  - ○ Self-critical thinking, catastrophize minor problems.
  - ○ Can develop delusions of guilt (psychotic symptoms discussed below).
  - ○ This negative style of thinking can progress to feelings of **hopelessness** (an important predictor of risk of suicide), **passive death wish**, and **suicidal ideas**.

Appetite, weight, and sleep disturbances are often grouped together as '**biological**' or '**somatic symptoms**', typically associated with **more severe** depression. Historically termed 'endogenous depression', it was suggested that this form of depression arose in the absence of any clear stressors, while 'reactive depression', seen as less severe, was usually a response to life events. It is more likely that these descriptions represent extremes on a spectrum of depressive events. Furthermore, while these 'biological symptoms' are associated with more severe depression in primary mental ill-health, they are very unhelpful in diagnosing depression in a medical setting, where patients often have these symptoms due to co-existing medical illness. Clinicians working in these settings are more reliant on '**cognitive**' **symptoms** (negative thoughts of guilt, hopelessness, self-criticism) (see Chapter 14).

6.2.2 Psychotic symptoms in depression

Psychotic symptoms **always** imply a more **severe** form of illness and must be documented. In mood disorders these are usually '**mood congruent**', i.e. the symptom is understandable in the context in which it arose. For example:

- Auditory **hallucinations** likely to be derogatory, critical voices.
- **Delusions**, often reflect the underlying depressive cognitions (see Table 6.2).

Clinical vignette Severe depressive episode

'Mrs S, a 56-year-old widow, was referred by her GP for OPD [Outpatient Department] assessment. She described feeling "awful", "living in a black hole". She had spent much of the previous two weeks in bed, unable to face the day. She couldn't sleep, lying awake, her head full of thoughts about the terrible things she had done in her life. She couldn't watch the TV or read the news, as she felt many

continued >

of the events reported were in connection to what she had done. She described feeling sad and low all day, worst in the morning time. She had lost her appetite, couldn't concentrate, had no interest in reading, or her garden, which she had previously loved. Even visits from her daughter did not cheer her up. Recently, she felt things would never get better and she would be better off dead. She said she would never harm herself but prayed every night that she would not wake up the next day. She had come to OPD very reluctantly as she did not feel anything would make a difference, but her daughter had insisted.' Community Psychiatrist

6.2.3 Other considerations

People may not experience all the symptoms presented in Clinical vignette Severe depressive episode. A patient who is depressed may not spontaneously disclose their symptoms and may need to be asked directly. In addition, some people may report feelings of anxiety rather than sadness.

6.2.3.1 Impact on function

Depression impacts on function in a variety of areas: work, home management (including family), private leisure, social leisure, and close relationships (see Isaac Marks, *Work and Social Adjustment Scale* for further reading). To diagnose any mental health disorder, there must be a negative impact on function. It is crucial to assess and document this—it will form part of treatment goals, as well as monitoring response. An assessment of the degree of functional impairment can be useful in making decisions on severity, but note that differences in baseline levels of activity occur between individuals, irrespective of the presence of depressive illness.

Table 6.2 Psychotic symptoms in depression (mood-congruent)			
Delusional beliefs in depression		Hallucinations in depression	
Subtype	Content (beliefs)	Subtype	Content
Guilt	Self-blame—untrue, excessive, inappropriate	Auditory	Derogatory, critical voices (*You are useless, worthless*)
Poverty	Are impoverished		
Hypochondriacal	Have serious physical illness		
Nihilistic (rare— occur in **severe** depression)	Have ceased to exist, or, in extreme form, parts of their body rotted away (Cotard's syndrome)	Olfactory	Unpleasant, repulsive smells Often explained by delusion, e.g. they are rotting away
Persecutory	People want to harm them, feel this is 'deserved'		

6.2.3.2 Depression and suicide

The lifetime risk of suicide in severe depression is up to 15%. Patients with depression can develop an increasing sense of **hopelessness**. This can be so severe that they feel life is not worth living and they may consider suicide. Patients who have lost hope are particularly at risk of suicide. Patients **must always be asked** about their hopes for the future and whether they have ever felt they cannot go on with life (see Chapter 2). Features in the history and mental state that are **particularly of concern** with respect to **suicide** include:

- Hopelessness—even in the most difficult of circumstances, most people retain hope.
- Thoughts (or plans) of self-harm.
- Signs that patients have made **advance plans**:
  - Putting their affairs in order (financial affairs, making a will, etc.).
  - Giving away things of value, e.g. their pets.
  - Writing a suicide note.
  - Taking extreme care in planning that they will not be found (choosing an isolated location, time when they are unlikely to meet anyone).
- Choosing and planning a method with **high lethality** (particularly violent methods, such as gunshot or hanging) or large amounts of a lethal substance (including medication).
- **Co-morbid mental illness**, particularly depression and schizophrenia.
- Social isolation, older age, male, family history of suicide.
- Other **vulnerability factors** include impulsive personality traits, history of childhood adversity, and presence of a chronic, painful illness.

These are **guiding statements** only. This is a complex area. With respect to the method chosen, for example, the patient's perception of lethality is important, even if the method itself is ultimately of low lethality. While a history of previous self-harm predicts further self-harm, identifying those who may go on to die by suicide is very difficult (see Chapters 15 and 18).

The presence of the above factors increases the level of concern about the patient and warrants early involvement of psychiatry teams in helping with the patient's care. If there is any concern about risk of further self-harm, **safe monitoring** of the patient is needed until a psychiatry assessment.

6.2.4 Diagnosing depression (ICD-10)

As with any mental health presentation, depressed mood can occur in other settings, particularly organic disorders. It is important to rule out any organic cause before diagnosing someone with a primary depressive illness. In general practice, up to 50% of patients with depression present with **somatic (physical) symptoms**, complicating the assessment.

European countries use the ICD-10 classification system (see Chapter 4). Depression is categorized either as a first or a recurrent episode (see Table 6.1).

A decision on severity is based on factors including the number of symptoms present: **mild** (four symptoms), **moderate** (five or six symptoms) and **severe** (seven or more symptoms). Clinically, differentiation rests on a complicated clinical judgement that involves the number, type, and severity of symptoms present. The extent of social, leisure, and work activities impaired is often a useful general guide to severity. It is very important to document the presence of **psychotic** symptoms.

Symptoms must be present **for at least 2 weeks** and should be present for **most of every day**.

6.2.5 Other clinical sub-groups

6.2.5.1 Recurrent depressive disorder

Two or more depressive episodes, separated by a period of time (months at least) where there was no evidence of depressive illness.

6.2.5.2 Atypical depression

Symptoms different to classical presentations:

- Increased appetite.
- Excessive sleeping.
- Mood, while depressed, is more variable and reactive.
- Marked anxiety.

6.2.5.3 Agitated depression

A depressive illness where agitation (purposeless restlessness) is prominent and severe. It is more common in older patients.

6.2.5.4 Seasonal affective disorder

A recurrent (atypical) depressive illness where episodes occur at the same time of the year (usually autumn/winter). There is a suggestion that it may be due to reduced hours of daylight. Treatments proposed include exposure to artificial light sources. Typical symptoms include excessive sleeping, increased appetite, with cravings for carbohydrates.

6.2.6 Demographics of depression

- Prevalence of 5–10% in the general population (higher in certain populations, such as hospital in-patients, prisons, nursing home residents, etc.).
- A leading cause of morbidity and mortality globally.
- More common in women—ratio of 2:1—this may represent under-reporting of depressive symptoms by men (more severe depression ratio nears 1:1).
- Average age onset: mid- to late-20s, further smaller spike in onset in later life.

6.2.7 Aetiology of depression

As with most mental illness, the underlying aetiology of depression is likely to be multi-factorial—an interaction between stressful events and underlying inherent vulnerabilities. A bio-psycho-social approach (see Chapter 4) is the most useful approach for the individual.

A summary of some of the theories are presented below to:

- Give you an introduction to the vast array of opportunities for further study and research in mental health.
- Allow you to focus your assessment to consider interventions.
- Help in education of your patient to understand their condition and how it may have arisen.

6.2.7.1 Aetiology of depression: biological theories

6.2.7.1.1 Genetics

Genetic studies indicate a role for inheritance, possibly by modifying individual response to stress (heritability rates for depression range from 40 to 70%).

6.7.1.1.2 Monoamine

Monoamine theory of depression suggests that depression is due to an abnormality in one or more of the monoamine neurotransmitter pathways (serotonin, dopamine, noradrenaline), either due to lack of availability of the neurotransmitters themselves or due to receptor abnormalities. Of these, **serotonin** (5HT—5 hydroxy-tryptamine) is the most clearly implicated. Evidence supporting their involvement includes:

- Anti-depressants either increase the release of monoamines and/or increase their availability by reducing their re-uptake (e.g. SSRIs).
- Abnormalities in neurotransmitter pathways or metabolites have been found in mood disorders.

6.2.7.1.3 Neuroendocrine hypothesis

This is an attractive hypothesis as it provides a biological explanation (activation of the neuroendocrine stress response) for the link between stressful events activating the physical stress-response (hypothalamic–pituitary adrenal (HPA) axis) and depression.

Evidence to support this comes from a variety of sources:

- The association of some endocrine disorders with mood disorders (e.g. depression in Cushing's disease).
- The presence, in depression, of abnormalities of the hypothalamic–pituitary–adrenal (HPA) axis, e.g. failure to lower cortisol levels in response to dexamethasone—abnormal dexamethasone suppression test (DST).

- The precipitation of manic symptoms by administration of exogenous steroids.
- Abnormalities of the immune system and depression (recent studies have focused on the immune system and depression, particularly the role of pro-inflammatory cytokines such tumour necrosis factor).

6.2.7.1.4 Structural brain changes and depression

These changes may be effects of depression rather than causes. Some suggest they may link to neuroendocrine theories, representing toxic effects of hypercortisolaemia, particularly on the hippocampus.

Consistent findings include:

- Enlarged lateral ventricles.
- Smaller hippocampal volumes.
- Reduction in grey matter in the pre-frontal cortex.
- In later life, increased white matter changes, associated with:
  O More severe illness, including neuropsychiatric symptoms such as apathy and impaired concentration.
  O Poorer response to treatment.
  O Co-morbid vascular risk factors.

6.2.7.2 Aetiology of depression: psychological theories

6.2.7.2.1 Cognitive theory

In the 1960s, Aaron Beck (a psychiatrist) proposed a novel way of looking at the negative thoughts associated with depression. He suggested that, rather than depression leading to negative thoughts, that negative thoughts led to depression. His treatment (**cognitive behaviour therapy**) sought to address and change these **negative thoughts**, which he divided into three different domains (**Beck's negative triad**):

- Negative views of oneself.
- Negative views of the world.
- Negative views of the future.

These patterns of thinking 'errors', **'cognitive distortions'** or **'unhelpful thinking styles'**, become the focus of treatment, aimed at treating and preventing depression (see Chapter 16).

6.2.7.2.2 Learned helplessness

In 1975, Seligman, a psychologist, noted that animals exposed to adverse events over which they have no control behave in a manner similar to the human experience of depression. They eat less, engage in less spontaneous activity, and, ultimately, fail to use opportunities to escape unpleasant situations. Seligman suggested that, in humans, depression occurs when consequences (positive or negative) no longer seem to depend on one's actions, i.e. there is a perceived loss of control over situations.

6.2.7.2.3 Psychosocial factors

In 1978, Brown and Harris, in a London study, identified four risk factors for the development of depression in women:

- Early maternal loss.
- ≥ three children under the age of 11.
- Unemployment.
- Lack of a confiding relationship.

While the validity of the findings remains under scrutiny, studies continue to examine these factors, more recently focusing on the role of a lack of a confiding relationship and 'burnout'.

6.2.8 Management of depression: general principles

Management only begins after careful consideration of the diagnosis, appropriate investigations, and construction of a biopsychosocial approach (see Table 6.3). Management will depend on the presentation:

- **Mild**, recent onset, no previous history—initial management may be monitoring with psychological support and education, family intervention, or social supports.
- **Moderately severe** will require either structured psychological intervention, such as CBT or drug treatment (see Chapters 16 and 17). Choice of treatment is guided by previous history of anti-depressant use, co-morbid medical conditions, medication, and symptoms.
- **Severe** depression (hopelessness, psychotic symptoms, poor self-care, lack of insight, and concerns re risk of suicide or, rarely, harm to others) may need admission, under the Mental Health Act (see Chapter 15) or ECT (see Chapter 17).

6.2.9 Course and prognosis of depression

- Between 65 and 75% of those treated for depression will have a successful response.
- On average, a depressive episode lasts about 6 months. The purpose of treatment is to reduce the duration of the episode and reduce the risk of recurrence.

Table 6.3 Diagnosis and management of depression general principles

Consider diagnosis	Consider aetiology	Grade severity and complexity	Match intervention to severity and causes
History, MSE	Biopsychosocial approach	Mild Moderate Severe	**Mild** Psychoeducation, behavioural activation, support
Differential diagnosis *Grief, adjustment, medical disorder,* e.g. ↓T4	Predisposing, precipitating, perpetuating factors	Psychotic features: Present Absent	**Moderate** Structured psychological treatments, e.g. CBT Anti-depressants, e.g. sertraline Educate, support, monitor Specialist referral if no improvement
Investigations* Collateral, physical, bloods, brain imaging, if appropriate	Use in planning interventions, e.g. family involvement, social support		**Severe** Urgent, specialist advice Consider anti-depressant (+/− antipsychotic) Crisis admission, if needed
			If concerned re risk of suicide seek specialist advice urgently

*See Chapter 4.

- Up to 60% of those who have an episode of depression may experience a recurrence.
- Proponents of CBT and related therapies suggest that the skills learned during these therapies help to reduce recurrence.

6.3 Bipolar affective disorder (BPAD)

Bipolar affective disorder (formerly known as manic–depression) is a major mood disorder in which the person can experience two extremes of mood: depressive (low) and manic (high) (or hypomanic—less severe) episodes (Figure 6.1). It is the presence of manic episodes that denotes the diagnosis of BPAD as, very occasionally, a person may only experience recurrent manic episodes. For many, the burden of illness is predominantly depressive episodes with infrequent manic episodes. As with depressive illness, the

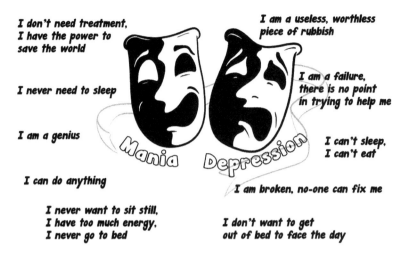

I don't need treatment,
I have the power to
save the world

I never need to sleep

I am a genius

I can do anything

I never want to sit still,
I have too much energy,
I never go to bed

I am a useless, worthless
piece of rubbish

I am a failure,
there is no point
in trying to help me

I can't sleep,
I can't eat

I am broken, no-one can fix me

I don't want to get
out of bed to face the day

Mania   Depression

Figure 6.1 Bipolar disorder—the two extremes.
© Eoin Kelleher.

presentation of bipolar illness can vary widely in terms of **severity, symptoms,** and the predominant **presentation**. As depressive episodes have already been presented, this section will focus on hypomanic and manic episodes. The depressive episodes of bipolar illness are diagnosed in the same way as those of unipolar depression.

6.3.1 Mania: core features

A manic episode (see Clinical vignette Manic episode) is characterized by **excessive and inappropriate elevation** in mood with an associated **increase in activity levels**. Clinical features include:

- Elevated mood—usually euphoric but can be irritable.
- Marked insomnia—often report a reduced need for sleep, different from the insomnia in depression when the person feels lethargic/fatigued.
- Racing thoughts with associated pressure of speech.
- Inflated self-esteem, grandiosity.
- Increased energy and marked distractibility.
- Behavioural abnormalities:
  o Socially inappropriate (disinhibition).
  o Reckless, e.g. over-spending, sexually promiscuous.
- Impaired insight—usually no recognition that the observed changes reflect illness.

Table 6.4 Psychotic symptoms in mania (rare)			
Delusional beliefs in mania		Hallucinations in mania	
Grandiose	Have special purpose or powers, or special connections, e.g. related to famous person	Auditory	E.g. hears voice of God speaking personally to them
Persecutory	People trying to harm them (less common)		

6.3.2 Hypomania: core features

Hypomania is a much less severe form of mania with minimal functional impairment and some insight.

6.3.3 Psychotic symptoms in mania

Psychotic symptoms in mania are rare, occurring in less than 20%. By definition, the presence of psychotic symptoms denotes a more severe form of illness. As with psychotic symptoms in depression, those that occur in manic states are generally **mood congruent** (see Table 6.4).

6.3.4 Manic stupor

(Rare), refers to catatonic features in an individual with a severe manic episode.

6.3.5 'Mixed' affective episodes

While some controversy remains about this presentation, occasionally people may present with a mixture of manic and depressive symptoms occurring at the same time, e.g. they may be overactive and pressured in speech but report predominantly negative thoughts. A person who experiences such episodes is still classified as having bipolar affective disorder.

Clinical vignette Manic episode

'A 20-year-old Brazilian student was brought to the Emergency Department by concerned friends. They said his behaviour had become increasingly irrational and impulsive. He had not slept for the previous three nights. He had arrived from Brazil eight months previously to study English. He was working in a bar every evening to support himself through college, frequently working until the early hours of the morning, and then getting up early to spend the day in college. In the ED he was overactive, pacing up and down the corridor, laughing to himself, speaking loudly. When interviewed, although he spoke excellent English, he frequently lapsed into Portuguese, speaking rapidly, switching from topic to topic, laughing frequently at "jokes" that were not understood by the interviewer. He explained that he had special talents that allowed him to predict the future of humanity and he wanted to share his ideas with the world. He also confided that he was related to Albert Einstein and was irritated when

continued >

this was questioned by the interviewer. He did not believe he was ill and was impatient to leave the ED as he planned to meet an investor to begin plans to communicate his ideas to the world. His urine toxicology screen was negative.'
Psychiatrist

6.3.6 Diagnosing bipolar disorder (ICD-10)
Diagnosis of a manic episode requires:

- A period of abnormally elevated mood with three or more symptoms of mania.
- Symptoms lasting at least 1 week (however, diagnosis can be made prior to 1 week if symptoms are severe and hospitalisation required).

An isolated episode (manic or hypomanic) is classified as below:

- Hypomania.
- Mania with psychotic symptoms.
- Mania without psychotic symptoms.

Bipolar affective disorder is only diagnosed when there have been at least two affective (i.e. mood related) episodes, one of which must have been a manic episode. It is the presence of mania (or hypomania) that dictates the bipolar diagnosis. Usually, one of these episodes is a depressive episode and the other is manic or hypomanic. Rarely, a person may present with recurrent manic episodes with no apparent history of depression.

6.3.7 Subsets of bipolar disorder (DSM-5)
- Bipolar disorder type 1 (mania and depression).
- Bipolar disorder type 2 (hypomania and depression).
- Rapid cycling—four or more episodes per year, fluctuating between mania and depression.

6.3.8 Demographics of bipolar affective disorder
- Prevalence of about 0.3–1.5%.
- Average age of onset is 21 years.
- In males, the first presentation tends to be with a manic episode; in females it is more likely to be a depressive episode.
- Male:female = 1:1.
- Affects about 60 million people worldwide.
- BPAD is associated with significant co-morbidity (particularly substance use and anxiety disorders).

- Rate of attempted suicide is up to 50% with about 10% of sufferers dying by suicide (more commonly during a depressive episode).

6.3.10 Aetiology of bipolar disorder

The concepts underlying aetiology in bipolar disorder are similar to those in depression. There is likely to be an interplay between stressful events and inherent vulnerabilities across biological, psychological, and social factors. As always, a structured, individual, biopsychosocial approach (see Chapter 4) is key.

6.3.10.1 Aetiology of bipolar disorders: biological theories

6.3.10.1.1 Genetics

- Genetic factors appear to play more of a role in bipolar than unipolar disorder.
- Heritability estimates of about 80% and monozygotic concordance rates of about 70%.
- The risk of **both unipolar depression and bipolar disorder** is increased in first-degree relatives of those with bipolar disorder.
- There is significant overlap in genetic risk factors between bipolar disorder and other mental illness, particularly schizophrenia.
- Children of those with bipolar disorder have a 50% chance of developing a mental disorder (schizophrenia as well as bipolar disorder).

6.3.10.1.2 Role of monoamines

It has been suggested that manic episodes may be secondary to excess dopamine. **Indirect** evidence for this includes:

- Manic states can be precipitated by dopamine agonists, such as bromocriptine.
- Stimulant effects of cocaine and amphetamine (both active at dopamine receptors).
- Medications that act as antagonists at dopamine receptors are beneficial in the management of manic episodes.

Serotonin and noradrenaline have also been implicated but their exact role is unclear. Serotonergic agents, such as anti-depressants, can precipitate mania (an important factor to consider when treating depression in those with, or at risk of, BPAD).

6.3.10.1.3 HPA axis and mania

As with depression, manic patients also display abnormalities in the dexamethasone suppression test and can have elevated levels of cortisol. Exogenous steroids can precipitate symptoms of mania (see Chapter 14).

6.3.10.2 Aetiology of mania: psycho-social causes

Mania was previously believed to be secondary to endogenous causes only. Although the association with life events is much more prominent in depression, at least some cases of mania may be precipitated be external factors- positive or negative events.

6.3.11 Management of mania: general principles

The principles of management of depression also apply here. Management only begins after careful consideration of the diagnosis and differential diagnosis, appropriate investigations, and construction of a biopsychosocial approach to allow a broad intervention.

There are some **important caveats**, however. Patients with mania rarely have insight into their illness, they frequently engage in impulsive and reckless behaviour, and are, therefore, unlikely to comply with treatment and likely to suffer significant adversity (as may others) early in their course. Furthermore, mania can deteriorate quickly. It is likely, therefore, that your role will be to assess, diagnose, and initially contain the situation, while seeking specialist advice.

Initial management (new presentation of mania):

- If on anti-depressants—stop them (they can precipitate and worsen mania).
- Start an anti-manic agent (antipsychotic), usually atypical, e.g. olanzapine or risperidone (better tolerated than typicals).
- Titrate dose according to response (**insomnia** is a useful monitor).
- If additional sedation needed, a short-acting benzodiazepine may be helpful (e.g. lorazepam) but please note this is symptomatic only, it has no anti-manic effect.
- If successful, electively seek specialist advice re subsequent management (e.g. length of time to maintain on medication).

6.3.11.1 Subsequent management

- If no/insufficient response, try another antipsychotic.
- Seek specialist advice/review, which is likely to include:
  - Addition of lithium or another mood-stabilizer, if not tolerated.
  - Admission.
  - ECT for severe, treatment-resistant mania.

6.3.11.2 Prophylaxis

Bipolar disorder (manic episode) has significant risk of relapse: 10–20% per year. Management includes life-style interventions, such as psycho-education, maximizing sleep, work, exercise, and social environments. Drug treatments, particularly mood stabilizers such as lithium, play a vital role (see Chapter 17).

6.3.12 Course and prognosis of BPAD

- Most patients recover from acute episodes.
- 90% of those who have had a manic episode will have a further mood episode, often with the intervals between episodes becoming shorter with time.
- As with depressive disorder, the more episodes a person has, the more likely they are to have another one.
- The average duration of a manic episode is about 6 months. The purpose of treatment is to shorten the duration of the episode and to reduce the risk of recurrence.
- Acute manic episodes will often require admission, as the patient frequently **lacks insight** into the seriousness of their illness. The association between mania and impulsive behaviour, such as over-spending, recklessness, and substance abuse, may make the patient **vulnerable** in an out-patient setting. Careful assessment is needed.
- Medication (including antipsychotic medication and mood stabilizers) is an essential part of treatment and is discussed in Chapter 17. As bipolar disorder is often a life-long condition, personal and family support and psycho-education are important components of management.

6.4 Other mood-related disorders

6.4.1 Dysthymia

- Chronic, low-grade depressive symptoms, not severe enough to meet a diagnosis of a depressive episode.
- Can develop superimposed episodes of depression.
- Prevalence about 5%.
- Female:male = 2:1.
- Can follow a chronic course, difficult to treat, often requires specialist intervention.

6.4.2 Cyclothymia

- Frequent episodes of mild depression and mild elation, not severe enough to meet a diagnosis of BPAD or recurrent depressive disorder.
- Prevalence 3–6%.
- More common in first degree relatives of those with BPAD.
- Chronic course.
- Symptoms may become severe enough to warrant a diagnosis of BPAD.
- Usual treatment is with a mood stabilizer, such as lithium.

6.5 Summary

Mood disorders comprise a significant proportion of mental illness. Presentations include depressed states, manic states, and a combination of both. The aetiology is still unclear, reflecting a complex interaction between underlying vulnerabilities and stressful life-events. Management requires a careful assessment of biological, social, and psychological factors, and will often combine medication with a psychological approach, such as CBT.

CHAPTER 7

Psychotic disorders

CHAPTER FOCUS

What you should know about psychotic disorders
- What does 'psychotic' mean.
- How may psychotic symptoms present in medical illnesses.
- How do you diagnose schizophrenia.
- What factors contribute to the aetiology of schizophrenia.
- What are the main drug treatments for psychosis.
- Do psychological factors play a role.
- What is meant by schizo-affective disorder and delusional disorders.

7.1 Introduction

The term '**psychosis**' is often misunderstood. It can be considered an 'umbrella-term' for symptoms that suggest the individual is unable to distinguish between what is real and what isn't, e.g. believing things that cannot be true (delusions) or seeing or hearing things that are not there (visual or auditory hallucinations) (see Glossary). It is, however, the **context** and **pattern** of these symptoms that define the underlying diagnosis. In 'true' psychosis (e.g. a primary **psychotic disorder** such as schizophrenia), psychotic symptoms, occurring in clear consciousness, are the **core features**, impairing behaviour, thought, emotions, and function. Other mental illnesses can include psychotic symptoms, e.g. severe depressive or manic episode with psychotic symptoms. In the latter, however, the primary pathology is the mood disorder; the psychotic symptoms, evidence of illness severity, and are usually 'mood-congruent', i.e. in keeping with the prevailing mood.

However, people can also experience isolated **psychotic symptoms** in other, often medical, settings—'organic' or 'physical' conditions, such as delirium or dementia (see Table 7.1). While these patients have isolated psychotic symptoms, they are not 'psychotic'—the primary process is not a psychosis. The underlying physical illness is driving the psychotic (and other) symptoms and this must be the focus of intervention.

Finally, adding to the confusion, the term 'psychosis' can be inappropriately used: e.g. in Korsakoff's 'psychosis', a disorder of memory impairment and confabulation, where there are rarely, if ever, any psychotic symptoms; Intensive Care Unit (ICU) 'psychosis', which seems to refer to a delirium (and occasionally post-traumatic stress disorder (PTSD) symptoms) in the context of an ICU admission; and steroid 'psychosis' where the patient is manic but rarely psychotic.

Table 7.1 Examples of psychotic symptoms in medical illness

Delirium (acute confusional state)	Hallucinations (usually visual) Delusions (paranoid ideas, occasionally delusional)
Dementia	Delusions (paranoid ideas, occasionally delusional) Hallucinations (visual, e.g. Lewy-Body dementia)
Epilepsy	Hallucinations (e.g. olfactory in temporal lobe epilepsy)

These distinctions are important. Incorrectly framing the diagnosis may hamper investigations and management. It certainly leads to miscommunications with medical and surgical colleagues who may view a patient as 'psychotic' when the underlying issues require urgent medical assessment and intervention. The (secondary) psychotic symptoms need adjunctive, symptomatic management (and support from psychiatry).

As noted above, this chapter will focus on psychotic symptoms in the context of primary psychotic disorders: schizophrenia, schizo-affective disorder, delusional and related disorders. Psychotic symptoms in the context of other illnesses are discussed in the relevant chapters. (Please see Glossary for explanations of terms).

7.2 Schizophrenia

Schizophrenia is a diagnosis based on a constellation of symptoms and signs rather than one pathognomonic feature. The person typically presents with **disorders of perception, thinking** and, in some cases, '**negative symptoms**' (see Table 7.2; Figure 7.1). It is usually characterized by faulty reality testing, manifest as delusions and hallucinations. These, in turn, lead to significant impairment of function across many domains (work, social, and personal) (see Clinical vignette Chronic schizophrenia).

Table 7.2 'Positive' and 'negative' symptoms of schizophrenia

'Positive' symptoms (presence of specific symptoms)	'Negative' symptoms ('absence'/loss of important features)
Delusions	Apathy—loss of motivation
Hallucinations	Blunted affect—little or no emotional response
Disorders of thought form	Anhedonia—no sense of pleasure, unlike depression, not concerned by this
	Attention—reduced
	Alogia—reduced spontaneity/quantity speech
	Social withdrawal—not distressed by this

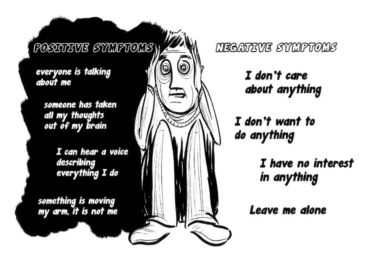

POSITIVE SYMPTOMS

everyone is talking about me

someone has taken all my thoughts out of my brain

I can hear a voice describing everything I do

something is moving my arm, it is not me

NEGATIVE SYMPTOMS

I don't care about anything

I don't want to do anything

I have no interest in anything

Leave me alone

Figure 7.1 'Positive' and 'negative' symptoms of schizophrenia.
© Eoin Kelleher.

As with many disorders, schizophrenia varies in severity and presentation, and probably reflects a group of heterogeneous disorders that share some characteristics. Some people experience infrequent psychotic episodes with recovery between episodes, others experience frequent and severe psychotic episodes with limited recovery.

Clinical vignette Chronic schizophrenia

'Mr S, a 54-year-old single man, attending community psychiatry, first presented in his early twenties, brought in by ambulance to the ED acutely distressed, agitated, shouting at [unseen] voices. He was convinced people were following him, trying to control him. They had begun to control his thoughts and had arranged for information about him to appear on TV. When alone, he could hear the voices commenting [negatively] on everything he did. He repeatedly tried to leave the ED to "get" the people who were plotting against him. He required rapid tranquillization and admission under the Mental Health Act. He responded to treatment with an antipsychotic and was discharged 4 weeks later. Over the next few years, he had several [similar] relapses, often precipitated by cannabis abuse and/or omitting his antipsychotic medication.

'Now, he had minimal acute symptoms. Instead, he spent much of his time in bed, on his own in supported accommodation. He had no interest in structuring his day, socializing or pursuing any form of employment. He had very poor self-care, and was frequently dishevelled. While, on questioning, he still

continued >

had persecutory delusions and occasional auditory hallucinations; these did not seem to bother him. He had gained significant weight and had developed Type 2 diabetes.' Community Psychiatrist

7.2.1 Clinical features of schizophrenia

Increasingly a '**prodromal**' period, the '**at-risk**' **mental state**, is recognized. The person has not yet developed acute psychotic symptoms but is exhibiting a change in behaviour (social withdrawal, loss of interest, vague, and preoccupied).

Positive symptoms (see Table 7.2) with lack of insight, are typical of the **acute phase**, manifest in disturbed thinking, muddled speech, and bizarre behaviour (withdrawn, overactive, or both). Over time, positive symptoms may become less, and negative symptoms, such as self-neglect and social withdrawal, become the most prominent features of **chronic** schizophrenia, often the most functionally disabling and most resistant to treatment (see Practical tips The six 'A's' of 'negative' (absence) symptoms in schizophrenia).

Practical tips The six 'A's' of 'negative' (absence) symptoms in schizophrenia

- Apathy—loss motivation.
- Attention—reduced.
- Alogia—reduced spontaneity, quantity of speech.
- Affect—blunted, little emotional response.
- Anhedonia—reduced or no pleasure. Unlike depression, not concerned by this.
- Alone—social withdrawal—not distressed by this, derives little pleasure from socializing.

Positive symptoms can recur at different times over the course of a schizophrenic illness. They may have distinctive characteristics. A diagnosis of schizophrenia was previously made on the presence of these distinctive symptoms, described by the German psychiatrist, Kurt Schneider, as **(Schneiderian) 'first-rank' symptoms** (see Table 7.3). These symptoms were later found to exist in other disorders and are, therefore, not pathognomonic of schizophrenia. However, ICD-10 uses them and their presence is highly suggestive of the diagnosis.

Disorder of **thought form** also occurs, where the structure of thought deteriorates (loosening of associations) so that thought processes can be hard to follow. 'Poverty of thought' may reflect the patient's experience of 'thought withdrawal'.

7.2.2 Clinical subtypes of schizophrenia

In addition to the prodromal, acute, and chronic phases of schizophrenia described in Section 7.2.1, ICD describes clinical subtypes—a concept abandoned

Table 7.3 'First-rank' (positive) symptoms of schizophrenia

Symptom category	Subtype	Examples
Hallucinations (auditory)	Commentatory voices ('running commentary' on their actions)	*She's putting her shoes on, now she's tying the laces*
	Repeating thoughts after they have happened ('Echo de la pensée')	*I must remember to do the shopping* (echoed after the thought)
	Speaking thoughts aloud as they are thought (Gedanken lautwerden)	*I must remember to do the shopping* (spoken aloud as thinking)
	Arguing or speaking about them in the 'third person'	*Look at him, he is a mess*
Delusions (of thought alienation or interference)	Thought insertion	*Thought in my head that isn't mine, was put there*
	Thought withdrawal	*My mind went blank, someone took my thoughts away*
	Thought broadcasting	*The people in the street know what I am thinking*
Delusions of passivity	Emotions, impulses, actions, bodily sensations under control of external force	*Look at my arm, it's moving but I am not moving it, someone else is*
Delusional perception	A 'normal' perception is interpreted delusionally	*The traffic light changed to green and I realized that the external forces were coming to power*

by DSM-5 as up to 80% of episodes present with features of paranoid schizophrenia. The terms are still used in ICD-10 and may be referred to in clinical practice.

Table 7.4 summarizes the four main subtypes. In **undifferentiated schizophrenia**, the person does not meet the full criteria for any of the subtypes described in the table or meets criteria for more than one subtype.

7.2.3 Diagnostic features of schizophrenia (ICD-10)

ICD-10 diagnostic features:

- Consciousness and cognitive function maintained (may be subtle neuropsychological deficits).
- Symptoms present for the majority of time ≥ 1 month.

Table 7.4 Clinical subtypes of schizophrenia (ICD-10)

Type	Paranoid	Hebephrenic	Catatonic*	Simple
Features	Most common	Child-like, disorganized, speech, behaviour	Disruption of muscle tone, movements	Slow, persistent decline in work and social function
Delusions or Hallucinations	Prominent, persecutory	Not prominent	Variable (state from stupor to excitement)	Not prominent
Onset	Older	Younger	Rare	Rare (difficult diagnosis)
Prognosis	Best	Poor	Poor	Poor

Catatonia* (profound psychomotor disturbance) can also occur in organic brain disorders (e.g. encephalitis) and severe depression and, as patients often refuse food and drink, is potentially life-threatening.

- Other causes of psychotic symptoms, e.g. drugs, mood disorder, excluded.
- Characteristic disturbance of thoughts and perceptions (**first-rank symptoms**—see Table 7.3)
- Not all patients with schizophrenia will exhibit first-rank symptoms. Other presentations include persistent, bizarre delusions (often persecutory in content), marked disorder of thought form (loosening of associations), and prominent auditory hallucinations.

7.2.4 Demographics of schizophrenia

- Point prevalence about 4 per 1000.
- Ratio of male: female 1:1.
- Usual age of onset—late teens, early 20s.
- Males earlier age, worse prognosis.
- Significant morbidity and mortality—about 20% reduction in life-expectancy.
- Increased rate of physical illnesses, such as cardiovascular disease, diabetes.
- Increased risk of suicide.
- Significant associated substance misuse (cannabis, nicotine).

7.2.5 Aetiology of schizophrenia

It is unlikely that any one mechanism will explain schizophrenia, given the diverse nature of its clinical presentation. Theories, with varying degrees of support, include the following.

7.2.5.1 Biological theories

7.2.5.1.1 Genetic

A genetic role is supported by evidence from family, twin, and adoption studies showing increased risk of schizophrenia, believed due to genetic rather than environmental factors. No single gene has been identified, rather a number of genetic abnormalities that additively confer susceptibility, interacting with environmental factors.

7.2.5.1.2 Neuro-transmitters and supportive evidence

Dopaminergic (DA) overactivity:
- Correlation between anti-psychotic medication efficacy and DA receptor blockade.
- Induction of psychotic symptoms by DA agonists (amphetamines, cocaine).
- Neuro-imaging studies.
- Raised plasma levels of DA metabolite homovanillic acid (HVA) and correlation with treatment response.

Serotonin (5HT): action of clozapine and LSD (a psycho-stimulant) on the 5HT receptor.

Glutamate: actions of ketamine and PCP on the glutamate-associated NMDA (n-methyl-D-aspartate) receptor.

GABA potential augmentation effects of benzodiazepines on anti-psychotics and some evidence of GABA-neuronal loss in the hippocampus of patients with schizophrenia.

7.2.5.1.3 Neurodevelopmental theories

Supportive evidence for the concept of schizophrenia as a neurodevelopmental (rather than neurodegenerative) disorder includes:

- Presence of cognitive and motor symptoms that **predate** the emergence of symptoms of schizophrenia.
- Excess of **obstetric** complications, e.g. low birth-weight, pre-eclampsia.
- **Neuro-imaging** studies suggest **structural** brain abnormalities at first diagnosis, post-mortem studies suggest these are without evidence of compensatory gliosis (scarring), postulating they may occur *in utero*.
- External markers of CNS dysfunction (dysmorphic and dermatoglyphic features).

7.2.5.1.4 Abnormalities in brain connectivity

Abnormalities in connectivity between fronto-temporal and parietal regions are documented by neuropsychological and neuro-imaging techniques.

7.2.5.2 Psycho-social theories

7.2.5.2.1 Family theories

Historically, several family-based theories were proposed to explain schizophrenia, including the concept of the 'schizophrenogenic mother' and abnormal family communication styles 'schism' and 'skew'. These were not supported by rigorous study. However, there is now substantial evidence from meta-analysis that experience of childhood adversity is associated with an increased risk of developing a psychotic disorder. Psychological and social factors may play a role in perpetuating illness, improving or worsening outcomes.

7.2.5.2.2 Social factors

The association between schizophrenia and lower socio-economic status seems to reflect **illness effect** ('downward drift') rather than causation. The high rates in urban settings and in immigrants could either reflect causation by stressful environments or differential migration due to illness. Premorbid schizoid personality is also a risk factor.

While this section (7.2.5) shows there is not yet clarity about causation, there are significant links between the aetiological theories and treatment strategies.

7.2.6 Management of schizophrenia

7.2.6.1 General principles

The management of a patient will be based on the outcome of a thorough and comprehensive assessment, to include consideration of the diagnosis, differential diagnosis, investigations, and construction of a bio-psycho-social approach (see Table 7.5). Due to the nature of the disorder, many patients may present with significant social adversity (homelessness, financial difficulties, lack of social supports), co-morbid substance abuse, or medical problems. These must each be assessed and managed appropriately.

The mental health intervention will depend on the nature of the presentation. Acute behavioural disturbance in the context of severe acute psychotic phenomena will require emergency intervention, medication, and may require admission (see Chapter 18).

7.2.6.2 Biological interventions

Anti-psychotics are the cornerstone of treatment (see Chapter 17).

7.2.6.3 Psycho-social interventions

Family and **psychological** (e.g. CBT):

- **Education** about symptoms and links with emotional and behavioural responses.
- Problem-solving strategies to manage symptoms.

Table 7.5 Diagnosis and management of schizophrenia: general principles

Consider diagnosis	Consider aetiology and management	Match intervention to individual presentation
History, MSE	Bio-psycho-social approach	**Psychological** Psycho-education (patient and family), CBT, family therapy
Differential diagnosis *Organic, e.g. substances (intoxication or withdrawal), epilepsy, brain disorders (encephalitis) Other mental disorders (acute transient psychosis, mood disorder)*	Predisposing, Precipitating, Perpetuating factors	**Biological** Anti-psychotics Benzodiazepines (acute presentation)
Investigations Collateral, physical, bloods, brain-imaging, EEG if indicated (consider metabolic effects), OT, social work	Use in planning interventions e.g. family involvement, social support	**Social** OT and medical social work (including work and finances)
	Regular monitoring of side-effects, physical health and response throughout treatment	Acute behavioural disturbance or risk of suicide seek specialist advice urgently

Social and occupational:
- Maximize social and occupational functioning.

7.2.6.4 Maintenance strategies

Schizophrenia will usually require life-long support, the nature of which will depend on initial response to treatment and severity of residual positive and, particularly, negative, symptoms.

Interventions, in addition to medication, will need to focus on **rehabilitation** for social and occupation functioning.

Depot medication, particularly where there has been a relapse while on oral medication, may be needed.

Monitoring for (and active treatment of) **emerging depression**, both in the acute phase and in the maintenance phase of the illness, is important. Depression can be difficult to diagnose in the presence of prominent negative symptoms (see NICE guidelines online) and is a significant risk factor for **suicide**.

7.2.7 Course of schizophrenia

Schizophrenia tends to be a persistent disorder:

- 1 in 5 recovers.
- 1 in 5 has persistent symptoms.
- 3 in 5 will improve but will relapse.

There are certain factors that can help predict outcome (see Table 7.6).

7.2.7.1 Factors that influence outcomes after diagnosis

7.2.7.1.1 Developing vs. developed countries

Evidence has shown that people with schizophrenia fare better in developing countries. The reasons for this remain unclear.

7.2.7.1.2 Life events

Life events can precipitate relapse of psychotic symptoms and worsen overall outcomes.

7.2.7.1.3 Family dynamics (the relationships between family members)

In a seminal paper in 1972, Brown, Birley, and Wing proposed that relapse rates were higher in people whose families showed 'high expressed emotion (high EE)' with the individual. By this, they meant families who were:

Table 7.6 Prognostic indicators in schizophrenia

Good prognostic indicator	Bad prognostic indicator
Sudden onset	Gradual onset
Short episode	Prolonged episode
No previous psychiatric history	Previous psychiatric history
Presence of mood symptoms	No mood symptoms
Persecutory subtype	Prominent negative symptoms
Female gender	Male gender
Older age at onset	Younger age at onset
Married	Single/separated/divorced/widowed
Good pre-morbid functioning	Poor premorbid functioning
No structural brain changes	Structural brain changes
Short duration untreated psychosis (DUP)	Long DUP

- Critical.
- Hostile.
- Emotionally over-involved (or enmeshed).

Further studies have confirmed the importance of these factors in relapse and outcome.

7.3 Schizo-affective disorder

This is a **rare** disorder in which the person has features of both schizophrenia and a mood disorder **present at the same time or within days of each other**—both sets of symptoms are equally prominent. Some believe that, rather than being a separate disorder, it exists on a spectrum between mood disorders and schizophrenia.

7.3.1 Clinical presentation of schizo-affective disorder
Three subtypes:

- Manic (similar in presentation and prognosis to BPAD).
- Depressive (more similar to schizophrenia).
- Mixed.

7.3.2 Management of schizo-affective disorder
Is based on principles of treatment for schizophrenia with additional management of the mood-related symptoms.

7.3.3 Course of schizo-affective disorder
- In general, the prognosis for schizo-affective disorder is better than for schizophrenia but not as good as that for mood disorders.
- Negative symptoms are rare.
- Prognosis is better for manic/mixed.

7.4 Schizotypal disorder

This is classified under schizophrenia in ICD-10 (and personality disorders in DSM-5). The person has some features of schizophrenia but delusions or hallucinations, if present, are fleeting or fragmented. With a prevalence of about 3%, it is more common in first-degree relatives of those with schizophrenia.

7.4.1 Clinical features
- Odd, eccentric behaviour.
- Idiosyncratic ways of thinking and speaking.
- Cold or inappropriate affect, social withdrawal.

- Transient, poorly formed ideas, including ideas of reference, magical thinking.
- Enduring symptoms, behaving more like personality disorder.

7.5 Delusional disorders

Delusional disorders are primary psychotic disorders in which the only (or main) feature is a **persistent delusional belief**. Other psychotic symptoms are absent or, if present, are fleeting and mild. There is no disorder of thought or speech. Over time, the delusion can become detailed and extensive.

7.5.1 Clinical presentation of delusional disorder

Depends on the content of the delusional belief. Personality is usually relatively well-preserved, but the person is usually very preoccupied with the belief and lacks insight. Some people may act on their beliefs—particularly those who are afraid or angry. Careful assessment, particularly with respect to risk, is important. Furthermore, because of the marked lack of insight, and often the single, focused delusion, these patients rarely present to psychiatrists, more commonly presenting to physicians (with physical symptoms) or lawyers (with paranoid beliefs). They are extremely difficult to treat, due to the fixity of their beliefs, the lack of insight, the poor response to antipsychotics, and the potential for risk (see Clinical vignette Delusional disorder).

Clinical vignette Delusional disorder (delusional parasitosis)

'The nurse in triage asked me to see the lady directly. It was her fifth presentation to the ED in eight weeks and she was concerned. I met the patient in a single room, accompanied by a nurse. A 52-year-old lady, she was agitated and distressed, somewhat dishevelled, with her hair askew. She initially was hostile and angry saying "what's the point, you won't believe me". She eventually agreed to tell me her story, a long and complicated one, which included a description of her microwave, which had stopped working eight weeks previously, which she had tried to fix and which she believed had released a gas that had caused insects to infect her skin. The insects were tiny, but she could see and feel them as they crawled around her skin. She had collected them in a matchbox, which she brought to the ED as 'evidence'. They made her feel 'itchy', uncomfortable, and afraid. Despite four trips to the ED, no-one had helped (or believed) her. She was considering taking a knife to burrow underneath her skin to dig them out. She denied any other symptoms. Her history, other than that she lived alone with poor social support, was otherwise unremarkable. The matchbox, which she held out for me to see, contained multiple bits of 'fluff' and tiny particles. She watched me carefully as I looked in, but I could see nothing that resembled an insect." Emergency Department Consultant

7.5.2 Demographics of delusional disorders

- Prevalence of about 0.03%.
- Average age of onset is 40s.
- Male:female = 1:1.
- Delusional jealousy is more common in men (**morbid, pathological jealousy,** or Othello syndrome).
- More common in women: **de Clerambaults** and **Capgras** syndrome.
- Depending on the subtype, better social and occupational functioning than those with schizophrenia; many are employed, some are in long-term relationships.

7.5.3 Specific delusional disorders

7.5.3.1 Delusional jealousy (Othello syndrome)

- Delusional disorder associated with the **highest risk of violence.**
- The individual irrationally believes that their partner is being unfaithful. Whether or not their partner is being unfaithful is not important, what is relevant is how they arrived at this belief. For example, they may believe their partner is being unfaithful because their neighbour's outside light is turned on at the same time every night.
- There may be accompanying beliefs, e.g. their partner is trying to harm them in some way.
- The behaviour that typically accompanies this belief of infidelity revolves around trying to find 'proof':
  - O Examining bedclothes or their partner's underwear for signs of sexual activity.
  - O Secretly following their partner to catch them in the act.
  - O Checking their partner's phone/computer, etc.
  - O Frequently confronting their partner demanding a confession (a false confession given to keep the peace only serves to exacerbate the situation).
- The person may or may not know who the supposed rival is.
- There is a **significant risk of violence** towards the partner and the supposed lover.
- There is also an increased risk of suicide.

7.5.3.2 Delusion of love (erotomania or De Clerambault's syndrome)

- The person believes that someone else, usually someone of a higher social status, is in love with them.
- There may not be any direct contact between them, but the person believes that their 'lover' is unable to contact them or to express their feelings directly.

- They infer expressions of love from innocuous or irrelevant comments or actions.
- Even explicit denials of love do not shake their belief and they can be persistent in their pursuit of the individual.
- This belief may take on a more persecutory and abusive tone when it may be associated with aggressive behaviour.

7.5.3.3 Capgras syndrome

- The person believes that someone close to them has been replaced by an imposter or double—the person may look the same, but they are in fact someone else.
- More common in women.
- Usually occurs in the setting of schizophrenia.
- May lead to aggressive behaviour towards the supposed imposter.

7.5.3.4 Fregoli syndrome

- The person believes that people who are strangers to them have been replaced by people they know—even though these strangers in no way resemble the people with whom they are familiar.

7.5.3.5 Delusional parasitosis (Ekbom syndrome), also known as delusional infestation

- Delusional belief that one's skin is infested with parasites.
- May have associated tactile hallucinations (formication), the feeling that parasites are crawling under their skin.
- Behaviour focused on gathering evidence of the bugs, often present with matchboxes filled with pieces of dead skin as 'proof'.
- Can occur as a primary delusion or secondary to agents that cause formication, such as cocaine or amphetamine abuse.

7.5.3.6 Induced delusional disorder (folie-à-deux)

- A shared delusional belief involving two people (more people may be involved but this is very rare).
- Usually, there is only one person who is truly psychotic, the other generally in a submissive relationship with the patient, heavily influenced by them, begins to take on the other's beliefs.
- The vast majority of cases involve members of the same family, typically in an isolated situation with little contact with the outside world.

7.5.4 Diagnosing delusional disorder (ICD-10)

- A single delusion or set of related delusions.
- Present for at least 3 months.

- Person doesn't meet criteria for schizophrenia.
- No persistent hallucinations.
- No prominent mood symptoms (or delusion persists even when the person is euthymic).
- No evidence of an organic disorder which would account for the symptoms.

7.5.5 Course of delusional disorders

- Variable.
- Better with:
  - ○ Shorter duration of symptoms.
  - ○ Jealous or persecutory subtypes.
- About **50% respond** to treatment (to varying degrees).
- The remainder have **persisting** symptoms.

7.5.6 Management of delusional disorders

- Difficult as majority have no insight.
- Risk of violence to self or others needs careful assessment. Admission to hospital may be necessary.
- Trial of anti-psychotic medication, although response often poor (about 50% respond). SSRIs have also been helpful (some overlap with OCD), but evidence is limited.
- Psychological intervention, including reality testing, support, and education.

7.6 **Summary**

While psychotic symptoms may present in isolation or in the context of other disorders, primary psychotic disorders are those where psychotic symptoms are the core features. This group includes schizophrenia (the largest contributor), schizo-affective disorder, and a smaller, less frequent group of disorders: delusional disorders, where the psychotic symptom is often restricted to a single, albeit elaborate, delusional belief system. Management is tailored to the presentation.

CHAPTER 8

Anxiety and obsessional disorders

> **CHAPTER FOCUS**
>
> What you should know about anxiety disorders
> - How to **recognize** pathological anxiety.
> - An understanding of how anxiety disorders **evolve** and links between disorders, such as panic disorder, phobias, and generalized anxiety disorder.
> - How to recognize post-traumatic stress disorder (PTSD).
> - An understanding of treatments for anxiety and stress-related disorders.
> - An appreciation of how anxiety disorders may exacerbate, co-exist with, or be mimicked by, **physical** disorders.

8.1 Introduction

Everyone experiences anxiety—it is part of normal experience. Anxiety **disorders**, however, are disabling conditions. In anxiety disorders, the person experiences severe, often persistent (or recurrent) anxiety that is excessive and/or inappropriate to the situation. It often co-exists with other psychiatric conditions (e.g. depression, substance abuse). In medical/surgical disorders, distinguishing 'normal' anxiety from an anxiety disorder requiring treatment can be very difficult. There are so many physical (bodily) symptoms of anxiety that patients often, understandably, believe they have a serious physical illness. This chapter will begin (as one does in clinical practice with patients) by explaining the physical (and psychological) symptoms of anxiety. A logical explanation, for what are often terrifying experiences, is the first step to helping the patient.

8.2 Key components of anxiety

See Practical tips Components (of all) anxiety disorders.

8.2.1 Physical and psychological symptoms of anxiety

Physical and psychological symptoms of anxiety are common (see Table 8.1). In anxiety disorder, these **physical** symptoms are severe and are then interpreted in a fearful way. Patients **believe** they are 'having a heart attack' or a 'stroke', are going to collapse, or die. This worsens their anxiety, worsening their physical symptoms, and a 'vicious cycle' ensues.

Table 8.1 Physical and psychological symptoms of anxiety

Physical	Psychological
Increased blood pressure, heart rate, experienced as palpitations (feel heart beating faster/harder)	Sense of apprehension
Over-breathing, 'breathlessness', light-headedness, tingling sensations in fingers/toes and around the mouth	Poor concentration
Dry mouth, nausea, 'butterflies in tummy', diarrhoea	Anxious interpretations of the physical symptoms, leading to worsening of the anxiety state
Muscle tension, tremor, tension headaches	Anxious ruminations (repeated thinking/worrying about something without ever reaching a solution)
Urinary urgency and frequency	

8.2.1.1 Physical symptoms of anxiety: a helpful explanation for patients

Presenting with strong physical symptoms of anxiety is, in fact, evidence of an 'excellent' response by the body to threat (Figure 8.1). It is the manifestation of the body's primitive 'alarm' system—the 'fight-or-flight' response. This is entirely appropriate (and helpful) in response to an immediate threat (for primitive humans, perhaps, escape from a predator). It is entirely unhelpful if one is sitting at home considering leaving to do the shopping or facing an interview. It is initiated by the amygdala and the hypothalamus, and co-ordinated by the sympathetic nervous system. The subsequent release of adrenaline and other substances triggers physiological responses that prepare the body for action. Thus, the tremor, palpitations, elevated blood pressure, and dry mouth are the effects of sympathetic nervous system activation. The 'tingling' (paraesthesia)is a consequence of 'over-breathing', leading to excessive CO_2 loss, a corresponding respiratory alkalosis, and abnormal nerve conduction. **An explanation of these responses** (in simple terms) is a helpful first step for patients to manage anxiety, and can be a platform for launching a psychological intervention

8.2.2 Avoidance

Practical tips Components (of all) anxiety disorders

- Psychological symptoms.
- Physical symptoms.
- Avoidance.

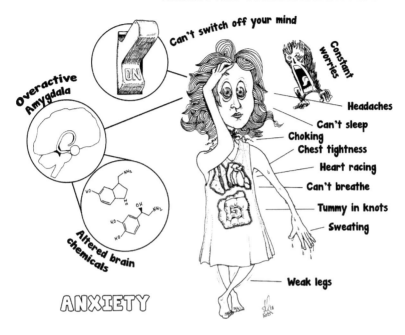

Figure 8.1 Clinical features of anxiety.
© Eoin Kelleher.

The vicious cycle between the physical and psychological symptoms of anxiety is a core part of the disorder. Avoidance is the next core response. Severe anxiety is an overwhelmingly unpleasant experience—patients become afraid of being afraid. They will do anything to avoid it. They begin to associate specific situations with anxiety and, as a result, avoid them. This leads to another vicious cycle, with the patterns of avoidance gradually increasing, so that some patients can become trapped in their own home.

8.3 Anxiety disorders subtypes: introduction

While the symptoms listed in Table 8.1 are central to all anxiety disorders, the patterns in which they present differ, which, in turn, influences treatment (and prognosis). The following sections discuss the various anxiety disorders and their management. We will start with phobias, as they are the easiest anxiety disorders to understand (and, often, to treat), then generalized anxiety disorder (GAD), hypochondriasis, and obsessive–compulsive disorder (OCD), ending with reactions to stress/trauma, including post-traumatic stress disorders (PTSD).

Note: There are many academic discussions as to whether OCD and PTSD should be considered anxiety disorders. For the purposes of this handbook, as they include prominent symptoms of anxiety, they are included here.

8.3.1 Anxiety disorders: shared key features

8.3.1.1 Aetiology

- Familial:
  - Often a positive family history, unclear if this is due to a **genetic** effect or to the family **environment**.
- Neurobiological:
  - The exaggerated autonomic response suggests possible neurobiological abnormalities (neurotransmitter or HPA) feedback dysregulation).
  - OCD has very specific biological links:
    - Specific response to serotonergic interventions.
    - Associated with PANDAS (paediatric autoimmune neuropsychiatric disorders).
- Cognitive:
  - Focus on physical symptoms promotes a vicious cycle of panic.
- Stressful events:
  - Precipitate, predispose (childhood), or perpetuate anxiety.

8.3.1.2 Co-morbid disorders

- Common:
  - Depression, other anxiety disorders, alcohol and substance abuse.

8.3.1.3 Treatment

- **Cognitive behavioural** strategies—helpful in many of the disorders.
- Drugs:
  - SSRI anti-depressants used for anxiolytic effects.
    - Serotonergic agents specifically helpful in OCD.
  - Benzodiazepines—powerful anti-anxiety drugs **but high risk of dependence.**

8.3.2 Anxiety disorders, a final general point: physical causes

Because so many of the symptoms in anxiety are physical, it is **crucial** to out-rule any underlying physical cause (see Clinical vignette Anxiety: physical cause and Practical tips Anxiety disorders). Possible causes include:

- Thyrotoxicosis.
- Phaeochromocytoma.
- Intermittent hypoglycaemia.
- Cardiac arrhythmia.
- Asthma.

Clinical vignette Anxiety: physical cause

'While I now work as a liaison psychiatrist, I initially trained in medicine, working in the ED on-call. A 64-year-old male self-presented, query panic disorder. He described recent onset of recurrent, brief episodes of over-whelming anxiety with a sense of impending doom. He would feel panic-stricken, unable to catch his breath, dizzy. He was now afraid to leave the house. Telemetry revealed intermittent heart-block [extract below] suggesting he was entirely correct to feel an impending sense of doom. He was referred for urgent cardiology assessment and pacing...

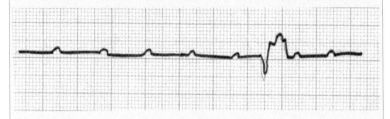

'There were a few "warning" features in the history—late-onset, male, and a history of dizziness. However, it was a stark reminder to me to **always** consider physical causes in "anxiety".' Consultant Liaison Psychiatrist

Practical tips Anxiety disorders

Always check for (and treat):
• Co-existing (comorbid) disorder, e.g. depression or substance abuse.
• Underlying physical cause.

8.3.3 Phobias
The key components of phobia are:

• **Fear** of an object or situation that is:
   ○ Irrational, extreme, or out of proportion.
   ○ Associated with **avoidance** (of the feared situation) that reinforces the anxiety.

8.3.3.1 Specific phobia
Specific phobias, previously termed 'simple' phobias, are associated with a specific situation or object (see Clinical vignette Spider phobia). There are many examples:

• Arachnophobia (fear of spiders).
• Fear of heights.
• Fear of vomit.

The **core features** are the same—overwhelming fear of a situation, leading to escalating avoidance.

> **Clinical vignette** Spider phobia
>
> 'Ms X, a 26-year-old female, described a life-long fear of spiders. "I was always afraid of spiders, but it has gotten worse. I realize it doesn't make sense. They terrify me. It's the way they suddenly scuttle towards you, you can't predict what they will do next." As a result, she avoided any situation where she might see spiders. She couldn't close her curtains at night in case a spider would fall out, she wouldn't put her hand into cupboards, wouldn't live in a basement, painted the walls of her apartment white, had white carpets (to make spiders visible). Gradually, the situations she avoided increased so that even the easiest of tasks frightened her. Most recently, she had found it difficult going into her local supermarket—the tops of tomatoes looked so like spiders she was afraid to walk through the vegetable section.' Clinical Psychologist

8.3.3.2 Additional features

- Females:males = 3:1.
- Prevalence 4–12%.
- Symptoms usually begin early (teens) (dependant on subtype).

8.3.3.3 Discussion

The vignette is typical of a specific phobia. This patient manages her fear by avoiding any situation that might cause it. While this initially leads to a reduction in fear, gradually the areas avoided increase. Clarifying the details is crucial. The patient is often relieved that someone understands them. Furthermore, it forms the structure for treatment (typically a combination of education and behavioural intervention, tackling the fears and avoidance).

8.3.3.4 Course and treatment

- Usually respond well to treatment.
- The treatment of choice is behaviour therapy (graded exposure) with psycho-education and cognitive strategies.

8.3.4 Social phobia

8.3.4.1 Core features

- **Fear**, excessive worry, about being judged, criticized by others.
- Physical and psychological symptoms of anxiety.

- **Avoidance** of any situation where this could happen (see also Clinical vignette Social phobia):
  - ○ Specific/performance type—fear of scrutiny in a specific situation (e.g. public speaking).
  - ○ Generalized (fear of scrutiny in most social situations).

Clinical vignette Social phobia

'Mr X, a 23-year-old college student, almost as soon as he left the house, would become anxious, feeling people were scrutinizing him. This would become worse when he was in a situation he couldn't escape (sitting on a bus, queuing in a shop, sitting in lectures). He knew his symptoms didn't make sense—not everyone could be judging him badly, but he was unable to conquer his fear. He had begun to avoid any social situations, only feeling happy to leave his house at night-time when no-one was around. Going to lectures had become impossible. He would feel anxious, his hands would start to shake, his palms become sweaty, sometimes he couldn't catch his breath. He felt his face would become flushed and red. Believing that everyone noticed these symptoms made his anxiety (and embarrassment) even worse. While he was not severely depressed, he had begun to feel increasingly low and desperate. He had started using alcohol to feel better, particularly if he needed to socialize, but felt worse next morning.' Psychiatrist

---

8.3.4.2 Additional features

- Equally common in males and females.
- Prevalence 2.5–13%.
- Symptoms usually early (teens) but may not present until much later.

8.3.4.3 Course and treatment

- Cognitive behavioural therapy (CBT).
- Anti-depressant (usually an SSRI) in severe cases or where they have failed to respond to treatment.
- Usually successful.

8.3.5 Panic disorder with and without agoraphobia

In panic disorder (without agoraphobia), the person experiences episodes of panic that are **not** situation-specific, occurring in a variety of settings, with no clear trigger (see Clinical vignette Panic disorder).

8.3.5.1 Core features

- Discrete episodes of intense anxiety/fear (physical and psychological symptoms).

- The psychological features are particularly catastrophic—**fear of dying, collapsing, or having a heart attack.**
- Last for several minutes (usually maximum of 30 min).
- Initially spontaneous, the patient has no awareness of what triggers the episodes.

Because, initially, the patient has no awareness of what triggers the symptoms, avoidance is not a key feature (other than avoidance of the distressing, fearful thoughts). Avoidance increases later, developing into agoraphobia.

Clinical vignette Panic disorder

'Ms Y, a 27-year-old lawyer, had recently experienced recurrent, severe, overwhelming panic. These episodes would come on without warning. She would feel dizzy, feeling unable to catch her breath, tightness in her chest, sweating, and shaking. During the attacks, she was convinced she would die. More recently, she had developed "pins and needles" in her fingers during the episodes, which convinced her she had heart disease. The attacks were now happening several times a week. She couldn't identify what was causing them and had begun to live in terror of when the next one might happen. She could not believe they were due to anxiety—they felt so "real". She was attending psychiatry out-patients, reluctantly, at the request of her GP.' Community Psychiatrist

---

8.3.5.2 Additional features

- Female:male = 2:1.
- Prevalence of 1.5–5%.
- Peak of onset mid-teens to mid-20s and mid-40s to mid-50s.
- The symptoms must be present for at least a month, with a minimum of four panic attacks over that time period.
- May be mimicked by other disorders (see Practical tips Other disorders to consider in presumed panic disorder).

Practical tips Other disorders to consider in presumed panic disorder	
Substance abuse disorders	Withdrawal symptoms mimic panic symptoms
Agoraphobia	In many cases, panic disorder has extended to include agoraphobia
NB Underlying medical disorders	Cardiac disorders (arrhythmias, mitral valve prolapse), hyperthyroidism, respiratory disorders (asthma, hypoxia), hypoglycaemia, phaeochromocytoma

8.3.5.3 Treatment

- CBT—including psycho-education, review of stressors/life-style.
- Anti-depressants (usually SSRI) if they have failed to respond to psychological treatment (see Practical tips Anti-depressants in panic disorder).

Practical tips Anti-depressants in panic disorder

NB Patients with panic disorder are very sensitive to the activating effects of SSRIs. Start at a **low** dose and increase **slowly**.

8.3.5 Agoraphobia

8.3.5.1 Core features

- Severe anxiety and panic.
- In situations from which escape may be difficult (e.g. crowds, public transport).
- Fear of collapsing/losing control/or having another panic episode.

Rather than risk losing control, and/or having an episode of panic, the person begins to **avoid any situation** from which they cannot easily escape. The avoidance can be so marked that the person becomes housebound.

8.3.5.2 Note

Agoraphobia can occur with (90%) or without (10%) panic symptoms. It has been suggested that an initial episode of panic triggers avoidance, gradually widening to include any environment away from home. Often the patient does not remember the initial episode.

8.3.5.3 Additional points

- Female:male = 3:1.
- Prevalence of 3–6%.
- Usual onset in 20s/30s.

8.3.5.4 Course and treatment

- CBT is the mainstay of treatment (graded exposure to the feared situations, cognitive strategies).

8.3.6 Generalized anxiety disorder (GAD)

8.3.6.1 Core features

- Worry—anticipation of (and plans to avoid) bad outcomes.
- Severe, excessive, intolerance of any uncertainty.

- **Differs** from other anxiety disorders by the **persistent** sense of apprehension and worried thoughts.

(See Clinical vignette Generalized anxiety disorder.)

Clinical vignette Generalized anxiety disorder

'Mrs X, a 58-year-old married lady, was recently diagnosed with breast cancer. She finished treatment, but still worried constantly with a feeling in the "pit of her stomach" that something awful would happen. She couldn't imagine returning to work (as a nurse). She couldn't sleep, lying awake at night worrying, couldn't concentrate, unable to make the simplest decision. She lost her appetite and was losing weight. She was particularly distressed and ashamed by her symptoms, berating herself for having "gotten through" her cancer treatment only to "collapse" now. Her oncologist told her all her tests were clear, yet she remained anxious, not about her cancer, about "everything". In retrospect, she thinks now she always suffered from anxiety but kept very busy, and never really focused on how she felt or thought.' Clinical psychologist

8.3.6.2 Additional points

- Female:male = 2:1.
- Prevalence of 2–6%.
- Onset in childhood and in later life.

8.3.6.3 Course and treatment

- Chronic, debilitating.
- Difficult to treat (about 30% remit after 3 years).
- Co-morbidities particularly important:
  - Alcohol abuse worsen prognosis.
  - Depression (suggested by the presence of early morning wakening and diurnal variation in agitation—worse in the mornings).
- CBT and 'third-wave', psychological treatments—mindfulness-based stress reduction (MBSR) and acceptance and commitment therapy (ACT).
- Anti-depressant (as anxiolytic), benzodiazepines (see Practical tips Benzodiazepines in anxiety).

Practical tips Benzodiazepines in anxiety

While benzodiazepines are very powerful anti-anxiety drugs, there are very significant risks of dependence.

8.3.7 Hypochondriacal disorder/hypochondriasis or illness anxiety disorder
Please see Chapter 14.

8.3.8 Obsessive–compulsive disorder (OCD)

8.3.8.1 Core features

- Obsessions:
  - Recurrent, intrusive, unwanted thoughts, images or impulses.
  - Person tries to resist them, does not act on them.
  - *'Home-made but disowned'*—recognizes they are their own thoughts but finds them abhorrent.
  - Typically, themes are particularly repugnant to the individual (see Clinical vignette OCD).
- Compulsions:
  - Behaviours (actions or thoughts) feels compelled to do.
  - Usually to prevent or 'undo' a negative outcome often (but not always) connected to an obsession.
  - Recognize action is illogical and senseless, tries to resist.
  - Does not get any enjoyment from the behaviour.
  - Carried out in a stylized, ritualistic manner.
- Typically patients present with both features but may present with mainly obsessions or compulsions.
- The clear link between the obsessions and the compulsions, and the sense of resistance, may be lost with time.

Clinical vignette OCD

'Mr X, a 42-year-old single man, had suffered all his life with unpleasant, distressing symptoms but was too ashamed to tell anyone. He constantly washed his hands, up to 20 times a day, taking 20 minutes each time. He had a particular routine, starting by washing up to his elbow, then washing his fingers, repeatedly, counting up to 20 each time. If he was interrupted, or lost count, he would have to start again. He used up to ten bars of soap a week. More recently, he had started to use bleach, scrubbing at his hands so that they were now red and sore, which is why he had presented to his GP. He was distraught about his symptoms, tired of washing his hands, tried hard to stop, but couldn't. Sometimes he would sit on the couch trying to stop himself from going to the sink. When he did this, his anxiety would get worse and worse until, finally, he "had" to do it. When he had finished, he would feel a little better, but only briefly. If he touched anything "dirty" he would immediately have to start again. More recently, the list of things that were "dirty" had gotten longer. He

continued >

wouldn't touch door handles, couldn't handle money, wouldn't shake hands. This was now "ruining" his life. He had stopped going out. The symptoms started in his 20s. Back then, he had been aware of fears of contamination, contracting a terrible illness from "bugs or viruses". But, more recently, he was so preoccupied by the behaviours that he had almost forgotten those thoughts.'
Community Psychiatrist

8.3.8.2 Typical obsessions

- Violent/sexual imagery or thoughts.
- Fear of doing something inappropriate/bad.
- Fear of contamination.
- Ruminations of doubt:
  o About **not having done** something (turned off the gas, locked the door).
  o Or **having done something** (*Did I hit someone while driving?*).
- Ruminations about decisions:
  o Endlessly weighing up the pros and cons of even minor decisions without ever coming to a decision.

8.3.8.3 Typical compulsions

- Checking behaviours.
- Counting.
- Handwashing/excessive cleaning.
- Need for symmetry (tidying or ordering).

8.3.8.4 Additional features of OCD

- Male = female.
- Prevalence of 0.5–2%
- Average age of onset late teens/early 20s (older at presentation).
- May occur in schizophrenia, anorexia nervosa, and physical disorders:
  o Basal ganglia disorders.
  o Sydenham's chorea.
  o PANDAS (paediatric autoimmune neuropsychiatric disorders associated with streptococcal infections)—OCD and tic disorder.

8.3.8.5 Course and treatment of OCD

- CBT:
  o Graded exposure (to feared situation) and response (compulsion) prevention.
  o Challenge exaggerated sense of responsibility, disprove harm predictions (behavioural experiments).

- SSRIs (and serotonergic tricyclic anti-depressant drugs (TCADs)), particularly where obsessions are prominent, patients cannot tolerate/fail to respond to CBT.
- Overall:
  - o 1/3 show significant improvement.
  - o 1/3 show some improvement.
  - o 1/3 show chronic symptoms.
  - o Symptoms often worsen/recur at times of stress.

8.4 Reactions to stress/trauma

In this group of disorders with prominent anxiety symptoms, it is assumed that symptoms only occurred because of the traumatic event.

8.4.1 Acute stress reaction

- Transient, **RAPID**, response to a significantly stressful situation (threat to life or security).
- Usually a mix of anxiety and depressive symptoms, fluctuate.
- The person may report feeling numb, having difficulty recalling what happened.
- Other symptoms may include agitation or aggression.
- No specific treatment. If the stress is removed then symptoms usually resolve within hours. If the stress continues, symptoms usually resolve within days.

8.4.2 Adjustment disorders

8.4.2.1 Core *features*

- **Gradual** response to stressful situation (see Clinical vignette Adjustment).
- Categorized according to predominant symptom-type (anxiety/depression/mixture of both).

Clinical vignette Adjustment

'Mr Smith, a 68-year-old widower, was brought to hospital by ambulance following collapse. He spent 10 days in ICU and had just been transferred back to the surgical ward. He was extremely distressed and anxious. He had fleeting memories of what had happened, describing a sensation of drowning, feeling he was dying. He remembered trying to fight with the attendants who were trying to help him, pushing away an oxygen mask. He was distressed, tearful, embarrassed, and frightened. As days passed, with support he could talk about his experiences and put them in context. Three weeks later his symptoms had almost gone and he was planning discharge home.' Pyschiatrist

8.4.2.2 Additional features

- Prevalence high in hospital (20%).
- Categories include:
  - Brief or prolonged depressive reaction.
  - Mixed anxiety/depressive reaction.
  - Predominant disturbance of other emotions/conduct.
  - Mixed disturbance of emotion and conduct.
- Symptoms arise within 1 month of the stressor and usually do not last more than 6 months.
- Precipitants include:
  - Physical illness, relationship breakdown, bereavement.

8.4.2.3 Course and treatment

- About 3/4 recover.
- About 1/5 have persistent problems.
- Treatment (usually CBT) tailored to symptoms:
  - Psycho-education, support.
  - Interventions to resolve the stressor (if appropriate).

8.4.3 Post-traumatic stress disorder (PTSD)

8.4.3.1 Core features

A significant, delayed response to a traumatic event related to death/threatened death/serious injury or sexual violation. Not everyone who experiences trauma develops PTSD. Individual vulnerabilities play a part. Of note, PTSD is no longer classified as an anxiety disorder in DSM, as themes of guilt, anger, and shame, as well as the presence of low mood, are recognized as significant issues in many presentations. There are three groups of symptoms associated with PTSD: symptoms of hyperarousal, re-living, and avoidance (see Table 8.2; Clinical vignette PTSD; Practical tips PTSD).

Table 8.2 Elements of PTSD		
Hyperarousal	**Re-living**	**Avoidance**
• Hypervigilance	• Flashbacks	• Emotional numbing
• Increased startle response	• Nightmares	• Avoidance of any reminders of event
• Sleep difficulty	• Intrusive imagery	• Feeling detached from others
• Irritability		• Difficulty recalling the event

Clinical vignette PTSD

'Mr X, a 32-year-old single farmer, abused alcohol. One night, after an evening spent drinking alcohol, he woke in the early hours of the morning, choking for breath. His room was filled with smoke. He couldn't see but could hear the crackling noise of flames outside his door and could feel intense heat coming through it. He heard crashing sounds like timbers falling and the sounds of windows smashing. He realized his house was on fire and was certain he was going to die. A neighbour raised the alarm and he was rescued by fire-fighters. He survived, but spent 3 months in the Burns Unit receiving treatment for extensive burns. He had no memory of his rescue.

'Six months later, he still felt constantly on edge, fearful something terrible would happen. His hands would shake, his palms were sweaty, his heart racing (physical symptoms of anxiety). He was unable to sleep, lying awake at night-time thinking about what had happened, fearful of nightmares where he was burning alive (psychological symptoms of anxiety). He would regularly feel he was back at the scene of the fire, could smell the smoke, hear crashing windows and falling timbers ("re-experiencing"). These "flashbacks" could happen spontaneously or might be caused by a sudden noise or smell that reminded him of the event. He was alert to any noise or sense of danger, easily startled by loud noises. He had become irritable, even with close friends, feeling "different" and "detached". While he re-experienced many of the sights and sounds of what had happened, he could not properly remember events, would become upset even trying to remember. He was unable to go back to his home or his farm, overwhelmed and distressed if nearby.' Clinical psychologist

8.4.3.2 Additional features

- Symptoms within 6 months of trauma.
- Female:male = 2:1.
- Prevalence about 8%.
- Risk factors: poor self-esteem, poor social supports, and history of mental illness or previous trauma.
- Co-morbid substance abuse, depression. and anxiety common.

8.4.3.3 Course and treatment

- CBT and EMDR (eye-movement desensitization and reprocessing).
- About 50% recover. Others follow a more chronic course.
- Post-traumatic presentations relating to **childhood** trauma or abuse typically require longer-term psychotherapy.

Table 8.3 Summary key concepts in anxiety disorders	
Understanding symptoms	
'Fight-or-flight' response	• A 'normal', automatic physiological response to threat, triggered inappropriately in anxiety
The 'fight-or-flight' response leads to	• Physical symptoms (sympathetic nervous system activation) • Psychological symptoms (catastrophic interpretation of the physical symptoms)
Avoidance response	• Acts to reinforce the fear and often leads to 'generalization' of the fear to multiple areas
Understanding causes	
Biological	• Genetics • Neurobiological abnormalities (HPA axis/serotonin)
Psychological	• Childhood experiences • Cognitive errors
Social	• Stressful events
Understanding treatments	
Behavioural (exposure) and cognitive strategies SSRIs	• Graded exposure to the feared situation • SSRIs particularly in OCD, also used for their anti-anxiety effect
Other features	
	• More common in women* • Often co-exist with other mental health disorders particularly substance abuse and depression • Remember to exclude underlying physical disorders, especially in panic disorder

* Exceptions are social phobia, OCD

Practical tips PTSD

'While PTSD is a complex disorder, remembering to construct the anxiety triad (PPA)—**physical** and **psychological** symptoms of anxiety, and patterns of **avoidance** is a good start in assessment. Additional features of re-experiencing, irritability and detachment, with strong feelings of guilt, anger, and shame mean these patients require expert psychological intervention by senior mental health professionals.' Clinical Psychologist, Hospital Medicine

8.5 **Summary**

This chapter on anxiety disorders has included a wide variety of disorders, including panic disorder, phobias, OCD, and PTSD. These disorders all share several common themes with respect to their symptoms, causes, and treatments (see Table 8.3). They are an important group of disorders to understand as they are common and, if untreated, very disabling for patients. As they often overlap with, or present to, medical settings, they represent a group that most healthcare workers in a medical setting are likely to encounter.

Eating disorders

9.1 Introduction

The core feature of eating disorders is preoccupation with:

- Food.
- Weight.
- Body shape.

This causes distress, functional impairment, and, often, physical as well as mental illness. The best-described eating disorders are anorexia nervosa and bulimia nervosa. More recently, binge-eating disorder has been described and an 'other' category, where features are not specific to one of the above diagnoses. This chapter focuses on the prominent disorders, anorexia and bulimia nervosa.

Clinical vignette Anorexia nervosa

'I cannot believe this young woman has an eating disorder but I suspect it is the case. She has attended my practice since childhood and is a capable lady, perfectionistic and a high-achiever, and recently started a demanding university course. I saw her 2 years ago when she was well, with a normal BMI. I was shocked by how emaciated she has become—slowed down, barely able to concentrate on the conversation. Her back was covered in fine, downy body hair. She had a low pulse (50 bpm) and blood pressure. She was unable to stand from squatting. Her BMI was 14.2 kg/m^2. She told me she was eating a "normal" diet. Closer questioning revealed this to consist of a black coffee for breakfast, an apple for lunch, and some chicken and vegetables for dinner in the evening, which she sometimes skipped as she felt "fat". Her periods stopped six months ago. I am very concerned about her. She is reluctant to attend for help.' GP

9.2 Anorexia nervosa (AN)

The diagnostic features of anorexia nervosa include:

- **Low body weight*** (self-induced, usually by restriction of intake, avoidance of 'fatty foods').
- Intense **fear of gaining weight**/pathological pursuit of thinness.
- **Distortion in body image** (the way in which one views one's weight or body shape), e.g. persistent denial of the seriousness of low weight, or belief that one's shape is abnormally fat.
- **Secondary amenorrhea** and/or reduced libido or impotence, or, if prepubertal onset, primary amenorrhea.

(See Clinical vignette Anorexia nervosa.)
***Weight** usually measured using the body mass index (BMI): weight (kg), divided by height (m^2). Normal BMI: 18.5–24.9 kg/m^2.
Reduced BMI can be subdivided into:

- Mild: BMI 17–17.5 kg/m^2.
- Moderate: BMI 16–16.99 kg/m^2.
- Severe: BMI 15–15.99 kg/m^2.
- Extreme: BMI <15kg/m^2.

Note: While absolute weight is a key indicator of severity, it may be the **rate of weight loss** (>1 kg/week) that is the urgent consideration. Some patients with AN can be 'stable' at a low BMI for many years.

Most patients with AN have **restricting sub-type**. They achieve weight loss through:

- Severe restriction of intake.
- Excessive exercise.

Occasionally, patients with AN may present with **binge-eating** and/or **purging** (self-induced vomiting, abuse of laxatives or diuretics). This form is **rare**, usually co-occurs with periods of severe restriction, and is distinguished from bulimia nervosa (BN) by **low weight** (in BN weight is usually normal, or increased) and the presence of other features of AN.

9.2.1 Additional features of anorexia nervosa

- Described in 1868 by William Gull (a physician), who focused on role of:
  - Weight gain.
  - Family.
  - Psychological causes.

Table 9.1 Anorexia nervosa physical and psychological complications

Physical complications		Psychological complications (difficult to distinguish from the effects of starvation)
Cardiovascular	↓BP, ↓HR, cardiomyopathy	↓concentration, ↓memory
Electrolyte/ Endocrine	↓K⁺, ↓glucose, amenorrhea	Reduced energy
Neuromuscular	↓muscle mass, proximal myopathy (inability to stand from squatting a key clinical sign of proximal myopathy), peripheral neuropathy	Social withdrawal
Haematological	↓Hb, ↓WCC, ↓Platelets	Depression
Dermatological	Lanugo body hair	Increased risk of suicide
Bone	Osteopaenia and Osteoporosis	Anxiety
Fertility	↓ (presumed due to weight-loss-induced abnormality of HPA axis)	Obsessive–compulsive behaviours often, but not always, associated with food (rituals associated with eating, e.g. eating in a specific order/specific food; occasionally other rituals, e.g. hand-washing)

- Female:male ratio of 10:1.
- Onset in adolescence.
- Recently, onset in pre-pubertal children and increased incidence in males.
- Serious medical and psychological co-morbidities (many secondary to severe, persistent, weight loss) (see Table 9.1)

9.2.2 Aetiology/associated factors
Aetiology is unknown. Associated factors include:

- Biological:
  o (Generally) emerges on a background of recent weight loss, usually, but not always, associated with dieting.
  o Genetic contribution supported by twin studies.
  o Biological abnormalities (HPA dysfunction), neuropsychological deficits, such as reduced concentration and attention, and some psychological features (depression and OCD behaviours) may be secondary to prolonged starvation.*

- *Psychological* (many speculative only):
  - O Family theories (enmeshment, over-protectiveness).
  - O Psychodynamic theories (fixation on the oral stage).
  - O Of note, however, is the consistent finding, first described by Russell and others, that family therapy is effective in the treatment of AN in patients under 18 years old. This therapy focuses on empowerment of parents managing the adolescent's behaviour, rather than any specific family-focused aetiology.
  - O Personality and temperament, driven at least partially by genetics (obsessional traits, especially perfectionism).
  - O Socio-cultural influences such as Westernization, media and social pressures.

*See **Minnesota Starvation Experiment**, a clinical study detailing physical and psychological effects of prolonged, severe starvation, many of which resembled features of AN.

9.2.3 Physical disorder
As with any mental illness, one must always consider an underlying medical disorder (e.g. malabsorption, inflammatory bowel disease). This is particularly important in the case of eating disorders when patients can present with 'unexplained' weight loss.

9.2.3 Course and treatment of anorexia nervosa
AN remains an extremely serious diagnosis with significant mortality (up to 15%), and morbidity. Of the remainder:

- About 1/3 recover.
- 1/3 achieve a partial remission.
- 1/3 continue with chronic AN.

9.2.3.1 Treatment includes

- Education and psychological support:
  - O Weight gain key, as many associated factors improve with weight gain. Slowed cognition at lower weight makes it difficult to engage in psychotherapy.
- Family therapy in the under-18 age group is the only consistently proven treatment method.
- Recent focus on early psychological interventions that incorporate support, education, and cognitive behavioural concepts. Examples include:
  - O CBT-E (enhanced cognitive behaviour therapy for eating disorders).
  - O SSCM (specialist supportive clinical management).
  - O MANTRA (Maudsley model of anorexia nervosa treatment for adults).

9.2.3.2 Hospital admission
In the presence of severe psychological or medical problems, or where outpatient treatment has failed, some patients will require hospital admission to stabilize their weight (see Practical tips Indicators for urgent medical admission).

> **Practical tips** Indicators for urgent medical admission
>
> These include:
> - Severe, rapid weight loss (>1 kg/week).
> - BMI less than 14.
> - Electrolyte disturbances.
> - Deterioration in physical complications, e.g. ↓BP, ↓HR.

Hospital admission will need to provide:

- Medical care (re-feeding).
- Psychological care.
- Psychotropic medication (rare).

9.2.3.2.1 Medical care—re-feeding

A key component of hospital admission will be the gradual introduction of food (re-feeding) with treatment of any physical or psychological problems. In-patient re-feeding must be carefully monitored and will require the input of senior medical consultants and clinical nutrition, as well as psychological support. Valuable guidance (*MARSIPAN—management of really sick patients with anorexia nervosa*), published by the Royal College of Psychiatrists, for hospital management of acutely ill patients with anorexia nervosa is available on-line (Figure 9.1). Careful teamwork is needed to manage these complex presentations (nurses, clinical nutrition, physicians, mental health teams).

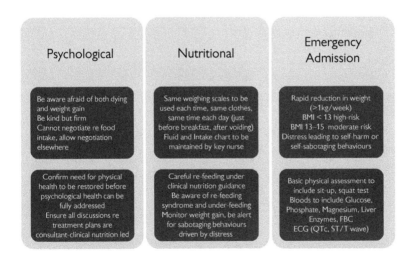

Figure 9.1 **Management strategies in medical care of anorexia nervosa.**
Source: Data from MaRSiPAN guidelines, Royal College of Psychiatrists.

Overly rapid correction of weight or electrolyte abnormalities may lead to fatal complications, such as gastric rupture or re-feeding syndrome. Re-feeding syndrome refers to severe metabolic disturbances with significant reductions in glucose, potassium, magnesium, phosphate, or thiamine. It probably reflects a shift in metabolism from using fat to carbohydrate, with corresponding increase in insulin release. Resultant shifts in electrolytes and fluid balance may precipitate heart failure, with reduced phosphate potentially leading to confusion, coma, or seizures. Expert clinical nutrition advice and careful monitoring and replacement of electrolytes and minerals will be needed.

9.2.3.2.2 Psychological care

Close team-work between physicians and mental health workers is essential in these complex presentations. An awareness that the person with AN is often as terrified of weight gain as of dying (if not more so) will make the medical carers alert for sabotaging behaviours driven by distress (Figure 9.1). A calm, clear, consistent, and firm approach is needed. Any major decisions will need to be taken at consultant level, and expert, consistent nursing input will be needed. The key message, that meaningful psychological work can only be done when the person is physically well-enough to engage, will need to be consistent. Evidence for the benefit of psychotropic medication in anorexia nervosa is scant, and this, coupled with the risks of side-effects in a significantly underweight, medically vulnerable patient, means that any prescribing should be done with care. Furthermore, some of the psychological effects, including poor concentration and low mood, are likely to remit as the starvation state is treated.

9.3 Bulimia nervosa (BN)

Clinical vignette Bulimia nervosa

'Anne initially seemed so cheerful—outgoing, chatty, no outward appearance of an eating disorder [normal weight]. But once I started to take the history, there were multiple problems—recurrent, "out of control" binges, making herself sick after every meal, packets of laxatives used every week, and a huge sense of self-loathing, guilt, and distress, a feeling that she was "ugly, fat, and unattractive" with alcohol her way to escape. She had finally come in after a serious overdose made her realize she needed help. She had been flagged on the system due to a low potassium.' Emergency physician

9.3.1 Diagnostic features
The diagnostic features of BN include:

- Recurrent episodes of **binge-eating** (defined as eating, in a discrete time-period, an amount larger than most would eat).

- A sense of **lack of control** over eating during these episodes.
- Compensatory behaviours to overcome binge episodes, including **purging** (self-induced vomiting and abuse of laxatives, diuretics, and other medications), or periods of fasting and over-exercising.
- As with AN, self-view is unduly influenced by concerns re **body shape and weight** (fear of fatness).
- Unlike AN, the patient with BN rarely reaches a low weight and is usually of normal, or slightly increased BMI.

(See Clinical vignette Bulimia nervosa.)

9.3.2 Additional features of bulimia nervosa
- First described (1979) by Gerald Russell as an 'ominous variant of anorexia nervosa' based on a case series of patients he had seen in clinical practice.
- Female:male = 10:1.
- Many are of **normal weight** and, as a result, usually have **normal menses**.
- May have history of AN.
- Multiple physical and psychological co-morbidities (see Table 9.2). Much more likely to have comorbid depression, anxiety, low self-esteem, and impulse control disorders, including impulsive self-harm (cutting or overdose), alcohol and substance abuse.

9.3.3 Aetiology/associated factors bulimia nervosa
- History of significant childhood adversity.
- Family history of substance abuse and/or affective disorder.

Table 9.2 Bulimia nervosa—physical and psychological complications

Physical complications* (*Many due to purging: self-induced vomiting or diuretic/laxative abuse)		Psychological complications
Electrolyte	$\downarrow K^+$, $\downarrow Na^+$, $\downarrow Cl^-$	Depression and anxiety
Gastro-intestinal	Dental erosions, parotid swelling, oesophageal erosions, oesophageal rupture, gastric ulcers, pancreatitis	Low self-esteem
Cardiovascular	Arrythmias, cardiac failure	Impulsive self-harm (cutting/overdose)
Haematological	$\downarrow WCC$	
Skin	Russell's pads (on fingers from putting fingers into mouth to induce vomiting)	Impulse-control disorders including alcohol and substance abuse

- As in AN:
  - O Onset usually in adolescence or young adulthood.
  - O May first occur in the context of dieting.
  - O Stressful life events also play a role.

Table 9.3 Typical features of, and differences between anorexia and bulimia nervosa*

	Anorexia nervosa	Bulimia nervosa
Weight	Low	Normal or increased
Intake (typically)	Reduced (severe, restricted)	Increased (binge-eating) with compensatory periods of restriction
Purging (Self-induced vomiting, laxative/ diuretic abuse)	Rare	Core feature
Preoccupied by weight and shape, fear of fatness, leading to distress	Yes	Yes
Amenorrhoea	Core feature	No
Body image distortion	Severe in context of emaciation	Less severe as weight often normal
Personality traits/ self-view	Perfectionistic, obsessional traits	Low self-esteem
Alcohol and substance abuse	Rare	Common
Physical Risks	Due to starvation, risk of death due to re-feeding	Due to electrolyte abnormalities (reduced potassium), oesophageal rupture and other effects of vomiting and purging
Treatment	Re-feeding, psycho-education, support, modified CBT	Psychoeducation, support, SSRIs, modified CBT, monitor electrolytes
Prognosis	Poor. Significant mortality (15%), 1/3 recover, 1/3 persist, 1/3 partial recovery)	Good. Majority do well (70%)

*Simplified version for students—patterns vary.

9.3.4 Course and treatment of bulimia nervosa

As severe life-threatening weight-loss is rare, the prognosis is generally much better than for AN. Majority (up to 70%) do well. Some persist with eating-related symptoms or issues with self-esteem.

9.3.4.1 Treatment includes

- Careful physical assessment, monitor electrolytes.
- **CBT** (for eating disorder and associated negative thoughts, low self-esteem, and mood).
- **SSRIs** (fluoxetine) may reduce the frequency of binge/purging.
- **Admission** rarely needed for physical problems but may be needed for severe depressive symptoms or self-harm.

While AN and BN are both eating disorders, there are significant differences between the two disorders with respect to their presentation, management, and outcome (see Table 9.3).

9.4 Summary

Eating disorders have become increasingly common and present in both medical and psychiatric settings. Anorexia nervosa is a serious, potentially life-threatening condition with a high mortality rate and is extremely difficult to treat. Bulimia nervosa, while less devastating with respect to mortality, can present with a variety of physical symptoms and significant psychological distress, low self-esteem, and impulsive behaviours, such as alcohol abuse and self-harm. Most healthcare workers are likely to encounter these disorders during their working lives.

CHAPTER 10

Psycho-active substance use

> **CHAPTER FOCUS**
>
> What you should know about psycho-active substance use
> - How to recognize alcohol dependence and prevent (or manage) withdrawal.
> - Consequences of alcohol abuse (physical and psychological).
> - Interventions to promote abstinence.
> - Consequences and management of heroin abuse.
> - Benzodiazepine abuse and withdrawal.
> - Newly emerging psycho-active substances.

10.1 Introduction

Psycho-active substance use, classified under mental and behavioural disorders (ICD-10), is categorized according to **substance** used and **presenting features** (see Table 10.1).

Each of these disorders varies, in severity and complexity, and according to substance abused. This chapter will focus on **alcohol**—the substance most commonly encountered in a medical setting. **Opiate** and **benzodiazepine** abuse will also be reviewed, with a final section on emerging patterns in drug abuse presenting to **emergency departments**.

10.2 Alcohol-related disorders

10.2.1 Recognition of harmful alcohol use

10.2.1.1 Taking an alcohol history

Taking an alcohol history (see Practical tips Alcohol dependency 'clues') is more than clarifying current dependency. It is an attempt to understand a person's relationship with alcohol and how it evolved. Like the structure for psychiatric history (see Chapter 2), the alcohol history follows a pattern related to the person's life.

- **Age** when first drink, drinking regularly, most days/every day.
- **Stressors** associated with increased intake.
- **Abstinence**—when, for how long, what helped?
- Current use:
  - What, where, when, with whom?
  - How do they pay for alcohol dependency?

Table 10.1 Mental and behavioural disorders due to psycho-active substance use—examples

Disorder	Substance	Presenting Features
Acute intoxication	Alcohol	Reflect substance used
Harmful use	Opioids	Damage to mental/physical health
Dependence syndrome	Cannabinoids	See Table 10.2
Withdrawal state (+/− delirium)	Cocaine	Symptoms on stopping/reducing substance. Indicates dependence
Psychotic disorder (+/− residual, late-onset)	Hallucinogens	Include hallucinations, ideas/delusions of reference
Amnesic syndrome	Alcohol	Marked impairment of recent memory

Source: Data from World Health Organization. (2004) . *ICD-10: international statistical classification of diseases and related health problems*, 10th revision, 2nd edn.

- **Harm** from alcohol:
  - ○ Health—physical/mental.
  - ○ Relationships.
  - ○ Employment.
  - ○ Finances.
  - ○ Forensic charges—pending/previous (drink-driving, public order, violence).
- **Treatments** (self-directed or result of family/court intervention)?
- **Family history** of alcohol or other substance use.

Practical tips Alcohol dependency 'clues'

People who are dependent on alcohol rarely volunteer or accept this. The following may suggest problem-drinking:

- Unexplained liver disease.
- Late onset seizures.
- Repeated, poorly-explained accidents.
- Psychiatric illness 'resistant' to treatment.
- Raised MCV.
- Raised gamma-GT.
- Conviction for driving while over the limit for alcohol consumption (rarely volunteered—always ask if alcohol abuse suspected).

10.2.1.2 CAGE questionnaire

The *CAGE questionnaire* does not diagnose dependence (Figure 10.1) but if a person answers yes to two or more questions, a more detailed history should be

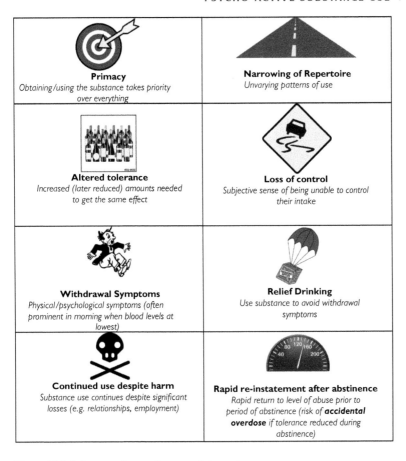

Primacy *Obtaining/using the substance takes priority over everything*	**Narrowing of Repertoire** *Unvarying patterns of use*
Altered tolerance *Increased (later reduced) amounts needed to get the same effect*	**Loss of control** *Subjective sense of being unable to control their intake*
Withdrawal Symptoms *Physical/psychological symptoms (often prominent in morning when blood levels at lowest)*	**Relief Drinking** *Use substance to avoid withdrawal symptoms*
Continued use despite harm *Substance use continues despite significant losses (e.g. relationships, employment)*	**Rapid re-instatement after abstinence** *Rapid return to level of abuse prior to period of abstinence (risk of **accidental overdose** if tolerance reduced during abstinence)*

Figure 10.1 Substance abuse—features of dependency.

taken. The use of an **'eye-opener'** suggests a high likelihood of **physical dependency** and risk of **withdrawal** states.

- Have you ever felt you should Cut down on your drinking?
- Have you ever been Annoyed by someone criticising your drinking?
- Have you ever felt Guilty about your drinking?
- Have you ever had an Eye-opener*? (A drink first thing in the morning to 'get going', often to overcome withdrawal symptoms, e.g. tremor, 'relief' use.)

10.2.2 Aetiology of harmful alcohol use

Likely to be multi-factorial, an interaction between the environment and individual vulnerabilities.

10.2.2.1 Biological theories

10.2.2.1.1 Genetics

A genetic contribution, possibly more prominent in men, is supported by twin (higher concordance rate in monozygotic (MZ, identical) versus dizygotic (DZ, non-identical) twins), and adoption studies. While genes that code for dopamine and GABA receptors have been implicated, no specific gene has been identified.

10.2.2.2 Psycho-social theories

10.2.2.2.1 Learning theories

- 'Learned behaviour' within the family.
- Dopamine-reward pathways motivate an individual to continue drinking.

10.2.2.2.2 Personality

- No specific personality traits—low self-esteem may play a role.
- Dissocial PD (with greater risk-taking behaviours) has a higher risk of substance abuse. However, most of those dependent on alcohol do not have dissocial PD.
- 'Locus of control' describes a person's sense of control over their own life. Those with an internal locus of control believe that they are 'in control'. They focus on finding solutions to problems they perceive as originating from their own decisions. Those with an external locus of control do not feel in control of their own lives, view their problems as originating from outside, and believe that there is little they can do to change the course of their lives. They tend to look to others to problem-solve, rather than taking personal responsibility. Some studies suggest 'external locus of control' is more prevalent in those with alcohol dependence

10.2.2.2.3 Social

- Societal average alcohol consumption influences rates of alcohol dependence. Ready availability of cheap alcohol is one factor but many other economic and cultural factors play a part.

10.2.3 Alcohol withdrawal

Always ask about previous withdrawal states and complications, e.g. seizures or delirium tremens. If present, the likelihood of complicated withdrawals during the current admission (unless managed) is high (see Clinical vignette Alcohol withdrawal).

Clinical vignette Alcohol withdrawal

'I had just started as an orthopaedic trainee. In the early hours of the morning I was called urgently to the orthopaedic ward. A young male, admitted 36 hours previously, was standing in the middle of the ward, dishevelled, tremulous, threatening staff and patients with a crutch (taken from nearby patient), hitting out at objects we couldn't see, shouting we were all out to get him. He ran out of the ward, down the corridor, and tried to get out of a [locked] window. I will never forget watching the patient try to smash the window to "escape". It took several staff to contain the situation and to administer appropriate medication. He had denied alcohol excess on admission, but on review had a clear history of alcohol dependency. I am now very clear that this is a preventable situation, one that is common in orthopaedic settings, and one we actively pursue.' Consultant Orthopaedic Surgeon

10.2.3.1 Alcohol withdrawal: clinical features

- Starts 4–12 h after last drink, peaks at 48 h.
- Usually lasts 2–5 days.
- Includes:
  - ○ Coarse tremor, nausea/vomiting, sweating, tachycardia, hypertension.
  - ○ Insomnia, agitation.
  - ○ **Seizures** (5–15%) peak incidence between 10 and 60 h after last drink. Increased risk if history of withdrawal seizures, co-morbid epilepsy, head injury, electrolyte imbalance.
- Delirium tremens (DTs):
  - ○ Severe form of alcohol withdrawal.
  - ○ **Physical** symptoms of both alcohol withdrawal and delirium.
  - ○ **Emergency**, if untreated, mortality rate of 10–15%.
- **Risk** factors include:
  - ○ Previous history of DTs.
  - ○ High levels of alcohol intake.
  - ○ Use of other psycho-active substances.
  - ○ Other physical/mental illness.

10.2.3.2 Alcohol withdrawal: management

Alcohol withdrawal is a **PREVENTABLE** condition: **identify** dependence and prescribe to **prevent** withdrawal (see Table 10.2).

10.2.4 Consequences of alcohol abuse

Alcohol abuse has widespread physical and psychological consequences (see Tables 10.3, 10.4).

Table 10.2 Alcohol withdrawal prevention and management*

Benzodiazepine	Thiamine/Vitamin B1	Other
Long-acting, e.g. chlordiazepoxide	Often deficient (reduced intake, absorption)	Fluids as needed
Dose—reflects: • Symptom severity • Liver disease • Cross-tolerance with benzodiazepines	Prescribe parenterally initially, then orally	Anti-psychotic, e.g. haloperidol if psychotic symptoms (monitor carefully, risk of reduction in seizure threshold)
Reduce and stop (risk may worsen confusion)	Prevent Wernicke's encephalopathy, Korsakoff's syndrome	Anti-epileptics—if adequately managed should not be needed
*Consult your hospital policy.		

10.2.5 Maintaining abstinence from alcohol

10.2.5.1 Psychological interventions

10.2.5.1.1 Brief interventions

Brief interventions (providing information, encouraging personal responsibility) in opportunistic settings (ED or GP surgery) may be helpful in misuse but not dependence.

Table 10.3 Consequences of alcohol abuse

Physical		Psychological
Liver	Hepatitis, cirrhosis, portal hypertension	Anxiety, depression Note: alcohol is depressant, difficult to disentangle alcohol abuse and mood
Pancreas	Pancreatitis	Social Phobia common
Cognition	Wernicke's, Korsakoff's, ARD* (see Table 10.4)	Suicide, delusional jealousy (increased risk)
Pregnancy	Foetal alcohol syndrome Effects of alcohol in pregnancy Low birth weight, small head/ stature, thin upper lip, smooth philtrum, difficulties with learning, attention, co-ordination	Schizophrenia comorbid alcohol use (20%), increased risk of tardive dyskinesia
* ARD: alcohol-related dementia.		

Table 10.4 Consequences of alcohol abuse—cognitive impairment			
	Wernicke's	Korskaoff's	ARD*
Onset	Acute	Chronic	Chronic
Aetiology	Thiamine deficiency	Thiamine deficiency	Unclear (?thiamine def., ethanol neurotoxicity)
Pathology	Mammillary bodies, thalamus	Mammillary bodies, thalamus	White matter loss (esp. frontal)
Clinical features	Nystagmus, ophthalmoplegia, ataxia, disorientation	Clear consciousness, anterograde amnesia (new facts registered but cannot recall), confabulation (invents facts to cover gaps in memory), unconscious process	Visuo-spatial deficits, poor planning, organization
Management	Thiamine (parenterally initially) Abstinence from alcohol	Thiamine (parenterally initially) Abstinence from alcohol	Thiamine (parenterally initially) Abstinence from alcohol
Prognosis	Good if treated, poor if not (80% Korsakoff's, 15% death)	Poor: 1/4 improve	1/3 better, 1/3 same, 1/3 worse

* **ARD**: alcohol-related dementia.

10.2.5.1.2 Motivational interviewing

Prompts problem-drinkers to reflect on their relationship with alcohol and assess its effects on their lives. It requires the person to be ready for change, moving through several stages from 'pre-contemplation' (do not recognize a problem), to 'contemplation' (accept there is one), through to preparing for action (these concepts were first elaborated by Prochaska and DiClemente). Later stages include maintenance and relapse prevention.

10.2.5.1.3 Residential detox

With repeated failure to abstain in out-patient settings, admission to a residential unit may help to achieve abstinence away from the challenges of life.

10.2.5.1.4 Group interventions

Alcoholics Anonymous (AA) is a voluntary organization focused on self-help with the support of others, and life-long abstinence from alcohol (www.alcoholicsanonymous.ie). **Lifering,** a secular, voluntary organization focuses on self-help using CBT (www.lifering.ie). Al-anon and Al-Ateen (AA-based) are support organizations for **family** members of those engaging in problem-drinking.

10.2.5.2 Pharmacological Interventions

One of the key challenges for those who have stopped abusing alcohol is **maintaining abstinence**. Medication, with psychotherapy, can be helpful.

10.2.5.2.1 Disulfiram (antabuse)

Disulfiram blocks acetaldehyde dehydrogenase leading to an accumulation of acetaldehyde when alcohol is consumed (Figure 10.2). This leads to an unpleasant reaction including:

- Facial flushing.
- Headache.
- Hypotension.
- Tachycardia.
- Nausea/vomiting.

Fear of the response can act as a deterrent. However, some individuals take alcohol while taking disulfiram, which is potentially dangerous. It is **contraindicated** in cardiovascular disease.

Other agents include:

Acamprosate	Naltrexone	Nalmefene
GABA +	Opioid antagonist	Opioid antagonist
Reduces urge to drink	Reduces heavy drinking, best in early stages	Reduces heavy drinking, taken 'as required'

Baclofen, Ondansetron and Topiramate have also been used.

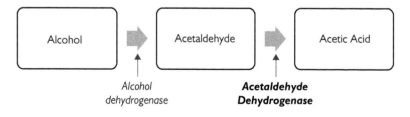

Figure 10.2 **Metabolism of alcohol.**

10.3 Opioids

Opioids refers to **agents that act on opioid receptors**, both naturally derived opiates (heroin, morphine) and synthetic agents (fentanyl, oxycontin). Prescribed opioids may be abused due to their euphoriant and anxiolytic effects, as may over-the-counter agents such as codeine. This section will focus on heroin abuse.

10.3.1 Heroin abuse

Initial euphoria diminishes as tolerance develops, with quick progression to **dependent** use, the focus being to avoid withdrawal symptoms (see Table 10.5).

10.3.1.1 Methods of use (powder—white or brown)

- Smoking.
- Snorting.
- Sub-cutaneous (skin-popping).
- Injecting.

It is rare for someone to start using heroin by injecting. If one is employing a **harm reduction** approach, then **avoidance of intravenous use** is one factor to address.

10.3.1.2 Consequences of heroin use

See Table 10.5.

10.3.1.3 Heroin withdrawal

- Unpleasant, distressing but rarely life-threatening.
- Symptoms begin 6 h after last dose and peak at 36–48 h:
  - Restlessness, cramps, rhinorrhoea, insomnia, sweating, diarrhoea, dilated pupils, tachycardia, piloerection ('goosebumps').

Table 10.5 Effects of heroin	
Desired effects	**Adverse effects**
Euphoria	Respiratory depression
Relaxation	Nausea/vomiting
	Constipation
	Loss of consciousness
	Effects of injecting: abscess, cellulitis, endocarditis, transmission HIV/HBV/HCV

10.3.1.4 Heroin withdrawal: management

- May be managed with symptomatic treatment (e.g. anti-inflammatories, anti-emetic, anti-diarrhoeal).
- **Methadone**—first-line (see 10.3.1.5.1).
- **Buprenorphine**, unlike methadone, is a partial rather than a full agonist at opioid receptors, thus it is less likely to lead to abuse or dependence. However, it can precipitate withdrawal as it competes with full agonists and has a higher affinity for the opioid receptors.
- **Suboxone,** a combination of buprenorphine and naloxone (opiate antagonist), means that any attempt to misuse buprenorphine by injecting it will precipitate withdrawal.

10.3.1.5 Opioid dependence: maintenance treatment

10.3.1.5.1 Methadone

- Opioid prescribed for withdrawal and maintenance, in individuals using heroin at high dose.
- Usually prescribed in addiction centres or specialist-GPs, identified on a central treatment list.
- If prescribing for an in-patient, check the dose with the prescribing centre first. Individuals may overstate heroin use due to fear of withdrawal. While withdrawal is not generally life-threatening, overdose is.
- Used as **maintenance therapy** with aim of **harm reduction**-minimizing harmful behaviours associated with heroin use. It may also facilitate engagement with services. Not all support this.
- Liquid form, starting dose is from 10 to 40 mg/day (1 ml = 1 mg).

10.3.1.5.2 Naltrexone

- Opioid antagonist.
- Theoretically may prevent relapse in stable, motivated patients.
- Rarely used.
- Some countries offer naltrexone (subcutaneous) **implants.** If a patient has a naltrexone implant, they will be **highly resistant to opioids for relief of pain,** requiring large doses of opioids with a risk of significant respiratory depression.

10.3.1.5.3 Therapeutic (group) communities

Focus on:

- Individual's substance-use and its impact.
- Interpersonal and social skills.

- Maintaining abstinence.
- Other members (and some staff) also substance users.

10.4 Benzodiazepine abuse

10.4.1 Dependence

- Occurs with longer-term use.
- **Iatrogenic** (i.e. long-term prescribing)—typically older women.
- **Illicit** typically younger adults, polysubstance abuse.
- Rapidly develop cross-tolerance and dependency on other benzodiazepines (BZDs), and alcohol.
- Taken orally, rarely injected.
- Use, especially in elderly, associated with increased risk of falls and cognitive impairment.

10.4.2 Benzodiazepine withdrawal

Benzodiazepine withdrawal can cause serious complications, particularly for hospital in-patients, when doses may be omitted, either because patients do not volunteer their use or, occasionally, doctors (correctly) judge that prolonged benzodiazepine use is inadvisable, but (incorrectly) judge that they should be stopped abruptly during their hospital stay. Presentations fall largely into two categories (see Clinical vignette The varied presentations of benzodiazepine withdrawal).

Clinical vignette The varied presentations of benzodiazepine withdrawal

'A 32-year-old man, admitted under the Mental Health Act with gross behavioural disturbance, had no known mental illness, but had recently decided to "stop everything" he abused. He was severely agitated, restless, aggressive, hitting out at staff, and punching the wall. His speech was incoherent and rambling. He appeared to be responding to auditory and visual hallucinations. He needed intensive nursing and medical input. He did not respond to high-dose antipsychotics. Collateral history suggested he had been heavily abusing benzodiazepines. Introduction of [very] high-dose diazepam, slowly tapered, ultimately contained his symptoms and behaviour.'

'Several months previously, a quiet, introverted 74-year-old lady had been admitted for surgery. Her post-operative recovery was complicated and she remained an in-patient for several weeks. On her third week of admission, she became increasingly aggressive and suspicious, with marked paranoid ideas. She also developed poorly defined visual hallucinations. Careful review of her history revealed that, unknown to staff, she had been on diazepam 5 mg bd for many years. Her symptoms resolved on re-introduction of diazepam.'

'Benzodiazepines, like alcohol, are common factors in presentations in acute hospitals.' Liaison Psychiatrist

---

10.4.2.1 Benzodiazepine withdrawal: symptoms and management
See Practical tips The RULE for benzodiazepine withdrawal.

Practical tips The RULE for benzodiazepine withdrawal

- <u>R</u>emember to ask (often forgotten).
- <u>U</u>nusual presentation (including psychotic symptoms), often delayed.
- <u>L</u>arge doses may be needed to treat (if abusing pre-admission).
- <u>E</u>quivalent doses of diazepam used and slowly withdrawn.

10.5 Emerging patterns of drug abuse

The patterns of drug abuse presenting to the ED are changing, influenced by several factors:

- Substances, particularly cannabis, cocaine, and methylenedioxymethylamphetamine (MDMA) (ecstasy), have increased in purity and potency.
- New psycho-active substances (NPS) developed to mimic the effects of controlled drugs and avoid legal controls.
- Poly-drug abuse.

10.5.1 Cannabis abuse

- Higher in males and younger adults (15–34 years) but increasing across all demographics.
- Around 1/5 classified as dependent.
- Long-term effects include poor memory, motivation, and mood, anxiety, and decreased ability to learn.
- Contains many different chemicals, the best known being tetrahydrocannabinol (**THC**)—largely responsible for the intoxicating effects of cannabis—and cannabidiol (**CBD**).
- Recent increased potency and higher THC content in cannabis has led to concerns about increasing rates of **psychotic disorder** across Europe (cannabis-use should be considered in an individual presenting with psychosis).
- **Withdrawal symptoms** include irritability, cravings, restlessness, insomnia, and anorexia. Cannabis can be detected for up to 28 days, depending on level of use and individual metabolism.
- **Intervention** includes motivational interviewing, CBT.
- **Short-term** hypnotics or sedatives may help withdrawal.

10.5.2 Cocaine

- Strong, short-acting stimulant extracted from cocoa plant.
- Inhibits re-uptake of neurotransmitters, including dopamine.

Table 10.6 Cocaine adverse effects	
Physical (sympathomimetic)	Psychological
Tachycardia	Anxiety
Arrhythmia	Hallucinations
Hypertension	Paranoid delusions
Hyperthermia	Suicidal ideation (especially in 'come-down' period)
Seizures	Dependence
Sudden cardiac death	Depression
Placental abruption	
Respiratory damage when smoked	
Risk of viral transmission sharing needles/nasal "tooters"	

- Usually sold as a powder, snorted, although it can also be smoked, rubbed on gums, or injected.
- Adverse effects (see Table 10.6).
- **Poly-drug** use common.
- Combined with **alcohol** produces cocaethylene—increases cardiac events.
- Injected with **heroin** ('speedball').
- Ketamine ('CK', 'Calvin Klein') increase in ED presentations (psychological symptoms).

10.5.3 MDMA (ecstasy)

- Methylenedioxymethylamphetamine, phenethylamine compound, weak hallucinogen, used for stimulant properties.
- Causes euphoria, increased sensory awareness.
- Emerged as a drug of abuse in the early 1990s associated with 'rave' music/dance, recently popular again with students in 'nightlife' settings.
- Usually taken as a **tablet**, a variety of brightly-coloured pills with different popular culture logos; can be obtained as a **powder** or **crystals**.
- Street names include Molly, Adam, Yokes, Buzzers.
- Potency increased recently.
- Slow-release preparations can lead to delays in the emergence of symptoms.
- Adverse effects (see Table 10.7).

Table 10.7 Ecstasy adverse effects

Physical	Psychological
Hyperthermia up to 41°C (can be life-threatening	Depersonalization
Arrhythmias	Hallucinations
Hypertension	Paranoid ideas, psychosis
Muscle-pain, jaw-clenching, restless legs	Agitation
Seizures	Disorganised thoughts
Sweating, flushes, water intoxication	

- **Treatment** focuses on the acute medical or psychiatric emergency, with referral to addiction services, if warranted.
- New substance 4FA (4fluoroamphetamine), 'ecstasy light', effects reported between those of amphetamine and MDMA.

10.5.4 Ketamine

- Dissociative anaesthetic and analgesic, 'club drug'.
- Approved use in medical and veterinarian setting, recently in resistant depression (registered specialists).
- Snorted, injected, or smoked.
- **High** doses cause dream-like states, altered consciousness, or hallucinations, can cause delirium, amnesia, impaired motor function, high blood pressure, depression, and potentially fatal respiratory problems.
- **Low** doses impaired attention, learning ability, and memory.
- Dissociative effect with amnesia may cause what is known as a **'K hole'**— the user has no recollection or awareness for a period of several hours.
- Other adverse reactions include severe vomiting, agitation, and bladder/urinary problems.
- A high **index of suspicion** should be present in situations at festivals where people present to emergency services with **vomiting and disorientation or memory problems**.
- **Methoxetamine** (MXE) called 'Rhino-Ket', side-effects more severe, include some opioid-like effects (respiratory depression), creatinine may be elevated.

10.6 New psycho-active substances (NPS)

- Manufactured to mimic effects of illicit drugs, sold as 'designer drugs'.
- Emerged on European market over past 12 years.

- Not controlled by International Drug Conventions but may cause a risk to health.
- Categories:
  - ○ **Synthetic cannabinoid** receptor agonists (spice products).
  - ○ **Stimulants or cathinones**: mephedrone, phenethylamines (crystal meth)—designed to mimic effects of traditional stimulants (cocaine, amphetamine), increased risk of suicide.
  - ○ **Opioids** (fentanyls) designed to mimic effects of heroin, much more potent than heroin, high risk of overdose.
  - ○ **iPEDs**—image and performance enhancing drugs includes steroids in bodybuilders and (injectable) tanning agents (melanotan). DNP (2,4 Di Nitro Phenol) is marketed as a 'fat burner'. Toxicity is high with this drug, which interferes with energy production at the mitochondrial level. Illicit vendors target chat rooms of vulnerable individuals.
  - ○ **GHB** (gammahydroxybutyrate):
    - Associated with 'chemsex' scene (methamphetamine, crystal meth, also used in this scene) where people use drugs to enhance their sexual experience.
    - A very narrow range between desired effect (1.5 mg) and overdose (2.5 mg).
    - Use was initially concentrated in the men who have sex with men (MSM) population but has become more mainstream in use within the last year.
    - Addiction a significant issue, withdrawal symptoms include severe agitation, hallucinations, seizures, and psychosis.
    - Treatment of withdrawals requires high-dose benzodiazepines, baclofen overseen by addiction specialists.

10.6.1 NPS: management

As with any case, the first step is to take a history and correctly ascertain what is being used. This can be more difficult that one might think (see Clinical vignette History in novel substance abuse). **Urinalysis** can determine up to 100 NPS when requested. Point of care tests (dipsticks) are available in most EDs and wards for immediate results. These screens usually cover the broad categories of opioids, benzodiazepines, cannabis, amphetamines, and cocaine. Some kits can also test for EDDP (methadone metabolite), 6-AM (heroin metabolite), alcohol, pH. **Synthetic cannabinoids and GHB** are **not** identified on routine screens.

Clinical vignette History in novel substance abuse

'I accompanied an experienced psychiatrist to a local clinic. He was convinced there were significant links between emerging novel substance abuse ("chemsex") and sexual health. The clinic's doctors had said there were no issues with drug abuse in their population. He sat in on the interviews and

continued >

noted that the question asked was, "Do you abuse drugs?". The answer was, invariably, "No". He suggested altering the question to: "Do you use drugs to improve your sexual experience?". The answer was, invariably "Yes, of course. Doesn't everyone?'.

'The experience taught me an invaluable lesson, one that recurs throughout clinical interviewing—the importance of adapting the questions to the interviewees.' Liaison Psychiatrist

Intervention focuses on the acute medical or psychiatric emergency, and discussion with addiction services when stable. The initial aim is to engage in brief motivational intervention.

10.7 Summary

Substance abuse presents to medical services in a wide variety of contexts. Histories are rarely volunteered and must be actively sought. Identification of substance abuse, and appropriate management, can prevent many clinical presentations. Specialist addiction services are primarily self-referral. Any intervention requires the person to be insightful into their substance use and take personal responsibility for change. Pharmacological agents are adjuncts to abstinence, supporting the significant psycho-social and lifestyle changes that an individual must undertake.

CHAPTER 11

Psychiatry of later life

11.1 Introduction

Psychiatry of later life (old age, psychiatry for the elderly) provides mental healthcare to older people with new-onset psychiatric illness (after age 65), and people with dementia complicated by behavioural and psychological symptoms of dementia (BPSD).

This chapter will discuss mood, anxiety, and psychotic disorders as they present in an older age group. It will begin with a review of **delirium** and **dementia**—challenging syndromes that frequently present to physicians. Basic assessment and management of these disorders should be familiar to all doctors. Psychiatry helps manage significant behavioural disturbance and more complex cases.

11.2 Delirium

ICD-10 describes delirium as: 'An etiologically non-specific, organic cerebral syndrome, characterized by concurrent disturbances of consciousness and attention, perception, thinking, memory, psychomotor behaviour, emotion, and the sleep-wake schedule. The duration is variable and the degree of severity ranges from mild to very severe.'

11.2.1 Delirium: clinical features and aetiology

See Figure 11.1, Table 11.1, and Practical tips Important points re delirium.

- An **acute onset** with marked **fluctuations** in severity (typically better during the day/worse at night), **disruption of sleep-wake cycle**.
- **Cognitive** deficits:
  - Attentional:
    - Inability to focus, shift, or sustain attention to external stimuli.
    - Distractibility—easily losing the thread of conversation.

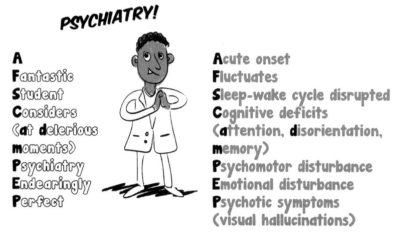

PSYCHIATRY!

A	**A**cute onset
Fantastic	**F**luctuates
Student	**S**leep-wake cycle disrupted
Considers	**C**ognitive deficits
(at delerious	**(a**ttention, **d**isorientation,
moments)	**m**emory)
Psychiatry	**P**sychomotor disturbance
Endearingly	**E**motional disturbance
Perfect	**P**sychotic symptoms
	(visual hallucinations)

Figure 11.1 Delirium: key features—a helpful mnemonic.
© Eoin Kelleher.

- Concentration poor (as demonstrated by serial 7s (see 3.2.6), months of the year, digit span).
  - Disorientation—temporal and spatial.
  - Memory impairment for new information, largely due to impaired attention (on recovery, patients often do not recall events).
- Psychomotor disturbance—typically agitation (hyperactive delirium), occasionally retardation (hypoactive delirium), or combination.
- Emotional disturbance, particularly lability but also perplexity, irritability, apathy, or indifference.

Table 11.1 Causes of delirium (mnemonic)	
Causes of delirium—key headings	Causes of delirium—mnemonic
Infection, e.g. UTI	I
Substances—intoxication (including prescribed drugs), side-effects, withdrawal	Suspect
Metabolic/endrocrine, e.g. renal, liver failure; hypo/hyperglycemia	Many
Intra-cranial infection, tumour, trauma	Interesting
Hypoxia (peri-operative, cardiac, respiratory)	Hypotheses

- **Psychotic symptoms,** including:
  - ○ Poorly formed persecutory **ideas** or ideas of reference.
  - ○ **Perceptual abnormalities** (illusions, hallucinations, typically visual)

Practical tips Important points re delirium

- Delirium **always** implies an underlying physical disorder.
- **Identify** and **treat** this disorder (see likely causes Table 11.1).
- Consider (often unrecognized) **pre-existing vulnerabilities,** e.g. cognitive/ sensory impairment, substance dependence, medical co-morbidities, older age.
- Advise on symptomatic management (environmental/medication).

11.2.2 Assessment of delirium

History and physical examination may be difficult. Cases often present at night when patients' teams are not available:

- Review the patient's notes/history, drug chart.
- Check **results** of recent physical observations/investigations.
- Seek **collateral** from nursing staff and family (where feasible).
- Be **alert** for any information that suggests underlying causes, e.g. marked tremulousness suggesting alcohol withdrawal.

Physical examination should be carried out if **safe to do so**. If not done, the reasons should be documented. Investigations are based on history and physical examination.

11.2.3 Management of delirium

The most important task is to find and treat the underlying cause. It can, however, take days (or sometimes weeks) for the person to return to baseline and symptomatic management may be necessary in the interim.

Environmental interventions can be very useful and may reduce or negate the need for pharmacological intervention. These include:

- A single, well-lit room with a clock and calendar to help orientation.
- Same staff to attend to the patient and family members.
- Ensure patient has glasses, hearing or other aids.
- 1:1 supervision.
- Mobilize as soon as possible, avoid 'naps' during the day.
- Psycho-education for staff and family.

Pharmacological interventions only if there is significant concern for **safety** of patient and/or others; if the patient is very **distressed;** and to facilitate **necessary**

Table 11.2 Medications in delirium

Antipsychotics*	Benzodiazepines
Usually first-line pharmacological treatment of severe agitation in delirium	First-line treatment if delirium due to alcohol or benzodiazepine withdrawal or if history of Parkinsonian symptoms
Haloperidol most commonly used. Olanzapine and quetiapine may also be used	Generally avoided, particularly in older patients (increase confusion and falls-risk)
Haloperidol can be given in PO/IM/IV forms	Older patients less able to metabolize BZD (particularly longer-acting forms) due to reduced hepatic function
Less likely to be associated with EPSEs when used short-term but monitoring essential	Short-acting forms such as lorazepam preferred (rapid onset, short half-life)
Majority of antipsychotics affect QTc—monitor ECG	

Please refer to your hospital guidelines for advice.

*Note:

1. Antipsychotics should not be prescribed in Parkinson's disease or dementia with Lewy bodies.

2. Antipsychotics (particularly atypicals) are associated with a greater risk of stroke and mortality in patients with dementia. As always, risks and benefits must be assessed before prescribing. Haloperidol has been used for decades but can cause extra-pyramidal effects in higher doses.

investigations/treatment. Careful consideration should be given to risks and benefits of treatment. Reasons for medication should be documented in the patient's notes.

In general, two groups of medications are used for the management of distressing symptoms of delirium: benzodiazepines and antipsychotics (see Table 11.2).

11.3 Dementia

Dementia is an **acquired, progressive, global** impairment of cognitive function, associated with significant social and occupational impairment. It typically includes memory impairment and impairment in at least one other cognitive domain. Features must not be explained by another mental disorder (e.g. depression) and must not only be present in the context of delirium, i.e. must **occur in clear consciousness**.

For a diagnosis of dementia, **ICD 10** requires impairment in two or more of the following **cognitive domains** (present for at least 6 months, causing functional impairment):

• Memory and learning (usually affected).
• Language.

- Executive functioning (planning/organising/evaluation).
- Perceptual-motor functioning.
- Social cognition.
- Attention.

Dementia is common, present in 5% of the community over 65, increasing with age to rates of 25–50% in those aged over 80 years. While most cases of dementia are irreversible, a **small percentage of cases are amenable to treatment**— a key initial step is to identify any treatable cause.

11.3.1 Dementia: presenting features

Dementia presents with **cognitive** and **non-cognitive** features (see Table 11.3), influenced by:

- Sub-type.
- Pre-morbid personality (possible exaggeration of pre-existing traits).

Table 11.3 Dementia presenting features			
Cognitive deficits (5 As)	Non-cognitive BPSD (behavioural/psychological symptoms dementia)		
Amnesia	Behavioural	Psychological	Physical
Attention	Agitation/disinhibition	Irritability/apathy	Nutrition—poor swallow/nutrition/weight
Aphasia	Wandering/restlessness	Depression/anxiety	Mobility—reduced/movement disorders
Apraxia^	Sleep-disturbance	Delusions/hallucinations	Seizures
Agnosia*	Poor self-care/social engagement		
Executive function#	Vocalizations (shouting)		

*Agnosia (difficulty recognizing objects despite intact perception).

^Apraxia (difficulty performing motor movement despite normal muscle function).

#Executive dysfunction—disruption of ability to 'oversee' cognitive processes, causing poor planning and judgement.

Note: 5 As—technically should be dyspraxia, dysphasia, etc. as use of the suffix 'A' suggests complete loss of function.

11.3.1.1 BPSD

- Present in up to 2/3 of patients with dementia.
- Major challenge to manage.
- Reflects:
  - O Brain-pathology (e.g. frontal—apathy, disinhibition, depression; temporal—delusions/hallucinations; basal ganglia—delusions).
  - O Environment.
  - O Psychological factors.

11.3.2 Dementia: aetiology

Dementia due to potentially reversible causes accounts for around 5% of dementia presentations and it is crucial to search for this when assessing patients (see Table 11.4).

11.3.3 Specific dementias: key points

See Table 11.5 and Clinical vignette Early Alzheimer's and fronto-temporal dementia.

11.3.4.1 Alzheimer's disease (AD)

- Commonest.
- Risk factors:
  - O Increasing age.
  - O Genetic—early onset: presenilin I and II, beta-amyloid precursor protein gene (chromosome 21); later onset: apolipoprotein E4 allele.
  - O Low IQ.
  - O Vascular.

Table 11.4 Dementia causes	
Reversible	Irreversible
Intra-cranial (tumour, subdural haematoma, normal-pressure hydrocephalus)	Neuro-degenerative disorders Alzheimer's disease (55%), Lewy body disease (15%), fronto-temporal degeneration (10% of early onset dementias e.g. Pick's), Huntington's disease, Parkinson's disease
Vitamin deficiencies (B12, folate, thiamine)	Vascular dementia (15%)
Endocrine (hypothyroidism, Cushing's disease)	Alcohol-related dementia
	Metabolic (Wilson's disease)

Table 11.5 Specific dementias—typical features

	Alzheimer's	Vascular	Lewy body	Fronto-temporal
Onset	Insidious	Acute	Variable	Younger
Decline	Gradual	Step-wise	Fluctuating, gradual	Gradual
Prominent symptoms	Amnesia (memory) (see 5 As)	Planning, sequencing, processing, attention	Parkinsonism, falls, visual hallucinations, variable cognitive impairment **Neuroleptic sensitivity**	Behaviour, personality Speech difficulties
Pathology	Atrophy—hippocampus, temporo-parietal, mainly cholinergic loss; plaques, neurofibrillary tangles	Multiple cerebral micro-infarcts	Diffuse Lewy bodies	Reflects sub-type, frontal/temporal regions

11.3.4.2 Vascular dementia

- Caused by cerebrovascular disease, often microvascular insults.
- Risk factors:
  - ○ Vascular.
  - ○ Genetic vulnerability (less common than in AD), e.g. 'stroke genes'.

11.3.4.3 Dementia with Lewy bodies (DLB)

Lewy bodies are abnormal intra-neuronal aggregations of ('normal') protein (alpha-synuclein); found in the brainstem in Parkinson's disease, but **throughout** the brain (cerebral/limbic cortex, hippocampus, midbrain/brainstem) in DLB.

11.3.4.3.1 Risk factors

- Gender—males.
- Family history of DLB or Parkinson's disease—no 'specific' genetic risks identified.

11.3.4.4 Fronto-temporal dementias

Previously termed Pick's disease, these are a group of neuro-degenerative conditions that typically present in **younger ages** (<65 years), with prominent behavioural/personality, motor, or language deficits, reflecting the underlying pathology (predominantly frontal/temporal). Sub-types include:

- Behavioural variant (impacts planning, judgement, empathy, socialization).
- Primary progressive aphasia.
- Disorders of movement.

Clinical vignettes Early Alzheimer's and fronto-temporal dementia

'I was asked to see a 67-year-old retired man in my GP surgery. He was brought in by his [concerned] wife. She had noticed he was increasingly forgetful—turning on the house-alarm at night, forgetting shopping [sometimes returning with nothing], regularly losing items like his car-keys. Twice, recently, he had forgotten where he had parked his car. He could no longer remember storylines of his favourite TV shows. He has no difficulty remembering distant events, and still enjoys life, eating well, gardening, and walking. He himself was aware that he was not functioning well and had difficulty with his memory.'

'The next patient was a 42-year-old man who presented saying he just "could not cope" any more. He could not explain it. Previously a quiet person, he found he was increasingly angry and irritable with everyone, losing his temper and shouting. He struggled to do simple tasks (using the oven, navigating on local transport, following conversations). He had stopped going to work (he worked as bank-clerk) as he could not do [previously "easy"] tasks. He was otherwise well with no significant medical history. He was concerned as one of his uncles had died from "dementia" aged 50 years.' Psychiatrist

---

11.3.5 Dementia assessment

Diagnosis is primarily based on:

- Careful history, examination (ideally in patient's own environment), i.e. **clinical judgement.**
- **Investigations** exclude potentially reversible causes and help define the likely site of brain pathology.
- **Collateral** history (as in all of psychiatry) is particularly important as patients may have little insight and BPSD, particularly challenging, must be carefully assessed.

11.4 Assessment of cognitive function

Assessment of patients' cognitive function occurs:

- During the **history.**
- At the **bedside**, using screening tests.

- If necessary, using more **complex neuropsychological tests**, usually carried out by expert psychologists.

Screening tools can be used both for assessment and monitoring.

11.4.1 Assessment of cognitive function (history) (patient/collateral)

- Education.
- Employment.
- Hobbies.
- Family-history dementia.
- Risk factors (e.g. smoking, history of vascular disease).
- Comorbid factors (physical or psychiatric illness).
- History of **onset** of symptoms, particularly cognitive features of dementia (four 'A's—Amnesia, Aphasia, Apraxia, Agnosia).

11.4.2 Assessment of cognitive function (bedside tests)
Level of arousal/**attention**:

- Orientation to time, place, and person.
- Spell WORLD forwards then backwards.
- Months of the year backwards.
- Serial sevens (subtract 7 from 100 and keep subtracting 7 from your answers).
- Digit span (remember up to six numbers forwards, four backwards). Choose a task that is in keeping with the patient's educational level.

Language (**aphasia**):

- **Speech:**
  - ○ Fluency, rate, spontaneity.
  - ○ Grammatical errors, neologisms (non-existent words) or paraphasias (unintended syllables or words in fluent speech), e.g. 'papple' for apple, 'lelephone' for telephone.
- **Comprehension** of commands (verbal/written):
  - ○ One-stage: 'Close your eyes'.
  - ○ Two-stage: 'Pick up the paper and fold it in half'.
- **Naming** (objects of increasing complexity, e.g. watch, strap, hand, winder).

11.4.3 Registration and short-term memory (amnesia)

- Ask patient to repeat three words (registration), distract them and ask to recall them after 5 min. (Impaired registration suggests deficits in attention; impaired delayed recall suggests damage to limbic structures.)

11.4.4 Specific bedside tests

Note: Many 'specific' cognitive tests invariably assess several functions simultaneously. For example, the clock-drawing test, often cited as a test of visuo-spatial/parietal lobe function, clearly also requires, amongst other things, comprehension of verbal commands, executive function (planning), and ability to co-ordinate muscular function.

11.4.4.1 4AT test

NB used primarily as a screening test for **delirium** but does give an indication of cognitive impairment.

- **Alertness** (normal/mildly sleepy/abnormal.
- **AMT4** (abbreviated-mental-test 4):
  ○ Age.
  ○ Date of birth.
  ○ Place.
  ○ Year.
- **Attention** (months of the year backwards).
- **Acute** change or fluctuating course.

11.4.4.2 MMSE (mini-mental state examination)

- Easy to administer.
- Scores of 23/30 or less suggest cognitive impairment.
- Not useful in mild cognitive impairment or frontal lobe deficits.

11.4.4.3 MoCA (Montreal cognitive assessment)

- More comprehensive than MMSE.

11.4.4.4 Clock-drawing test

Several versions. Tests variety of domains, including comprehension, planning, visuo-spatial ability, e.g. patient, given a sheet of paper, asked to 'draw a clock, put in all the numbers, and set the time to ten-past-eleven'.

11.4.5 Tests according to suspected area of pathology

11.4.5.1 Frontal lobe

Features suggesting frontal lobe pathology include:

- Personality change/disinhibition.
- Poor personal care/judgement.

11.4.5.2 Frontal assessment battery

- Short screening test of executive function.
- Helps distinguish **frontal**-type dementia from **Alzheimer's** type.
- Six parts:
  - Similarities/categories: 'how are orange and apple (chair/table; tulip/rose/daisy) the same?
  - **Verbal fluency** (name all the words that start with S in one minute—no place-names/names).
  - Motor series (**Luria test**) (imitate examiner first—hand in fist, then out-stretched on side, then palm down).
  - **Conflicting instruction** test (if I tap once, you tap twice; if I tap twice; you tap once).
  - **Go/no-go test** (if I tap once, you tap once; if I tap twice, you don't tap).
  - **Environmental autonomy** test (put your hand in mine and do not hold my hand).

11.4.5.3 Temporal lobe

Features suggestive of temporal lobe lesions include:

- Receptive (fluent) dysphasia (Wernicke's area)—inability to understand language.
- Verbal memory deficits.
- Proposagnosia (inability to recognize faces).
- Auditory hallucinations.

11.4.5.4 Specialist testing

Includes the **CAMCOG** (Cambridge cognitive examination) and the **ACE-R** (Addenbrooke's cognitive examination).

11.4.6 Risk assessment in dementia and older age

Usual concepts of risk apply to patients of older age, but with the addition of several other risk factors:

- **Risk to self**: self-neglect (personal/physical care), wandering/exploitation by others (e.g. financial or sexual).
- **Risk to others**: verbal/physical aggression, forgetfulness, e.g. forgetting about items on the cooker leading to a fire risk, sexually disinhibited be-haviour (uncommon), driving.

11.4.7 Management of patients with dementia

Treat any potentially reversible causes as discussed.

11.4.7.1 Management of BPSD

Non-pharmacological interventions are key:

- Identify challenging behaviour.
- Detailed description, contributory factors (pain, sensory impairment, etc.).
- Generate behavioural intervention, including meaningful recreational activities, one-to-one empathic engagement.
- Support care-givers.
- Maximize function.
- Reminiscence and multisensory therapy, cognitive stimulation.
- Pharmacological agents (including antipsychotics):
  o Avoid if possible.
  o Most useful in aggression and psychotic symptoms.
  o Associated with increased mortality, particularly vascular events.
  o Use for defined time, with regular review.
  o Lowest possible dose, increase slowly, monitor side-effects.

11.4.7.2 Management specific to the dementia

- Treat any comorbid psychiatric illness.
- Acetylcholinesterase inhibitors (ChEIs) and memantine slow progression of symptoms of dementia (see Table 11.6) and are used in both AD and DLB.
- For vascular dementia, manage underlying vascular risk factors.

Table 11.6 Agents used to help slow progression of symptoms of dementia			
Name of medication	Class of drug	Indication for use	Key points
Donepezil	2nd generation ChEI	Mild-moderate cognitive impairment	Long half-life, highly selective—less side-effects once-daily
Rivastigmine	2nd generation ChEI	Mild-moderate cognitive impairment	Short half-life safe in asthma and COPD twice-daily
Galantamine	2nd generation ChEI	Mild-moderate cognitive impairment	Short half-life twice-daily
Memantine	NMDA receptor partial agonist	Mod-severe cognitive impairment	

11.5 Specific features of mood and psychotic disorders in later life

11.5.1 Depressive disorder

Some features are more prominent in older patients:

- Psychomotor disturbance (agitation or retardation).
- Delusional themes are typically persecutory, nihilistic, or hypochondriacal.
- Higher risk of suicide.
- Physical complaints/worsening memory.
- Association with cerebrovascular disease (known as **vascular depression**' or 'depression-dysexecutive syndrome'), more likely to have deep white matter changes on neuro-imaging, more difficult to treat, more cognitive deficits.

11.5.1.1 Depressive pseudo-dementia

Presents with prominent subjective memory complaints but without clear-cut dementia—the apparent cognitive deficits are due to depression. In practice, it can be hard to distinguish the two (see Table 11.7), a situation further complicated by the fact that depression is common in dementia.

11.5.1.2 Treatment for depression later life

Similar to younger people. The SSRI anti-depressants are generally preferred due to their more favourable side-effect profile. QTc prolongation and hyponatraemia may occur. Older medications, such as TCADs, with marked anticholinergic side-effects, can be particularly problematic in an older population.

Table 11.7 Depressive pseudo-dementia and depression distinguishing features

Dementia	Depressive pseudo-dementia
Unaware of extent of deficits, rarely reports problems	Reports significant deficits, not supported by collateral history
Usually attempts to answer questions	Tends to give 'I don't know' answers during cognitive testing, reluctant to engage
Mood is usually normal but there can be varying distress	Pervasive and persistent low mood
Rarely exhibits guilt/worthlessness, suicidal ideas,	Guilt/worthlessness, suicidal ideas common
Gradual, progressive decline in higher cognitive functions; attention/concentration usually intact initially	Marked difficulty with concentration

11.5.2 Bipolar disorder

Mania presents as in younger patients, however, fluctuating disorientation and paranoid ideas can cause difficulties in diagnosis. Care must be taken when prescribing for older patients. **Lithium** (see Chapter 17) is used as a mood stabilizer but monitoring is needed and levels should be kept at the lower end of the therapeutic range (0.4–0.6 mmol/L). Some older adults may develop symptoms of lithium toxicity despite levels within 'normal range' (0.4–1 mmol/L). Long-term use is associated with increasing risk of nephropathy—reduction in estimated glomerular filtration rate (eGFR), increased renal indices. It may be necessary to switch to a renal-sparing agent, e.g. sodium valproate. However, the risk to physical health needs to be balanced with the risk of destabilization of mood in someone stable for years on lithium (seek specialist advice).

11.5.3 Psychotic disorders

It is rare, but possible, for a psychotic illness to present for the first time after aged 60-years. It is important to **out-rule an organic cause**, and to manage any reversible risk factors (sensory deficits, isolation). Late-onset psychosis is more common in women and more likely to present with delusions and hallucinations. Treatment is with low-dose antipsychotics. Side-effects (extra-pyramidal side-effects (EPSEs), tardive dyskinesia, Parkinsonism) are increased. Atypical antipsychotics less likely to cause EPSEs, are associated with increased risk of cerebro-vascular event (CVA). Always exclude Lewy body dementia before prescribing anti-psychotics.

11.5.4 Other presentations in later life

11.5.4.1 Senile squalor syndrome (Diogenes' syndrome)

This condition is **not associated with any one diagnosis**. It is characterized by severe neglect of self and surroundings, marked social isolation and resistance to all offers of help. The individual engages in extreme hoarding, a risk not just to themselves but also to neighbours and visitors (e.g. fire, attracting vermin, etc.) Exclude a primary mental illness (depression/psychosis/OCD), a neurodegenerative condition, particularly fronto-temporal dementia or response to stress in someone with a pre-morbid vulnerable personality.

In the absence of a major mental illness, public health legislation may be used to clear the property.

11.5.4.2 Charles Bonnet syndrome

The person experiences vivid, visual hallucinations into which they retain insight. There are no other psychotic symptoms and no evidence of an underlying delirium/dementia.

It is not a mental illness. It is most common in older people with visual impairment. Symptoms often improve if vision is restored or if it is lost completely. Education as to the cause of the hallucinations can reduce any associated distress and antipsychotics are not indicated.

11.6 Summary

With an aging population and increasing rates of hospitalization of elderly patients, it is important to know how mental illness presents in older patients. Delirium and dementia are common presentations. Knowledge of how to recognize and manage them is essential. An awareness of the impact of older age on both presentation and treatment of mental illness is also crucial.

CHAPTER 12

Child, adolescent, and perinatal psychiatry

CHAPTER FOCUS

What you should know about child, adolescent, and perinatal psychiatry
- Specific aspects of assessment and consent in children.
- Presenting features of common childhood disorders (neurodevelopmental, mood, and anxiety).
- Common risk factors and interventions in children/adolescents.
- Key features of mental health in pregnancy and childbirth.

12.1 Introduction

This chapter focuses on the impact of mental illness in children at all stages—directly (child and adolescent psychiatry) and indirectly (perinatal psychiatry). The chapter begins with childhood-related disorders. Children may develop mental illnesses as discussed in earlier chapters (depression, anxiety, eating disorders, etc.) This chapter provides advice re mental illness and:

- Assessing for mental illness in **children** (including consent).
- Specific disorders of childhood.
- Mental illness and childbirth.

12.2 Assessment

While assessment of children resembles that of adults, it is important to note that children often come to attention because of the concerns of **others** (e.g. parents or teachers). A more systemic approach is used, therefore, with greater emphasis on **developmental history** (usually from parents), **collateral history** (parents, school), and their **environment** (family, school, peers) (Figure 12.1). Assessment may include a school visit to observe behaviour outside the family environment, and usually includes more than one member of a multi-disciplinary team. As with adults, rating scales may be useful but should not replace a thorough assessment.

This reliance on others can cloud the picture—an overly anxious parent may seek help in the absence of mental illness. Conversely, a child in need may not receive help if their care-takers do not perceive a problem.

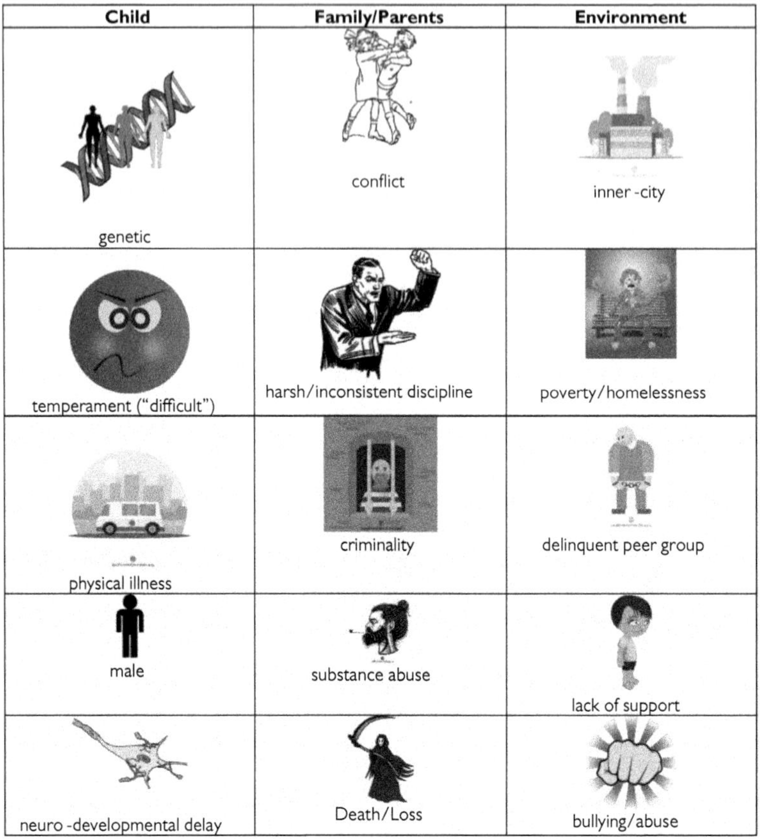

Child	Family/Parents	Environment
genetic	conflict	inner-city
temperament ("difficult")	harsh/inconsistent discipline	poverty/homelessness
physical illness	criminality	delinquent peer group
male	substance abuse	lack of support
neuro-developmental delay	Death/Loss	bullying/abuse

Figure 12.1 Children and mental ill-health—risk factors.

12.2.1 Interviewing

The approach depends on the age/development of the child. Usually, more than one session will be needed to gain understanding and develop rapport. As with adults, a common-sense approach is needed. Jargon or leading questions should be avoided. Sometimes alternative ways of communicating, e.g. through play or drawing, may be needed. Whether a parent/guardian is present during the assessment depends on the age of the child and their wishes (as appropriate). Older children may speak more freely if a parent is not present.

12.2.2 Consent

Under normal circumstances, consent must be sought from both parents before assessing any person under the age of 18. (This may vary in different jurisdictions.) Adolescents may be deemed to have the right to consent or refuse interventions, if judged to have capacity to make that specific decision ('Gillick' competence). Parents can also **refuse** treatment for a child. If this is felt to conflict with a child's best interests, application to the Courts may be made for a judicial opinion. It is clearly best to engage the child's consent.

12.2.3 Collateral from parents/guardians

Includes:

- Antenatal/postnatal complications.
- Developmental milestones.
- Medical history.
- Premorbid personality.
- Family history, including family dynamics (bearing in mind that information provided may not be an objective account).
- The problem for which help is sought and how it evolved.

Accounts given by members of the same family may differ. This can help illustrate family dynamics.

12.2.4 School—information

Includes:

- Peer/teacher relationships.
- Academic functioning.
- Observed emotional or behavioural problems, including variation between home and school, people present.

Classroom visits can be helpful but are not always necessary.
Brief rating scales for specific disorders may also be included.

12.2.5 Physical examination

Includes:

- Overview of physical health.
- Any evidence of congenital disorder.
- Height, weight.

- Neurological exam.
- Other investigations, if indicated (e.g. baseline ECG or bloods prior to psychotropic medications).

12.3 Neurodevelopmental disorders

These are characterized by abnormalities in development of the central nervous system. Examples include autism spectrum disorders and attention deficit hyperactivity disorder (ADHD). Other **developmental learning disorders** include specific delays in reading (dyslexia), writing, maths, or motor coordination (dyspraxia), generally presenting in childhood and improving with age and support, and tic disorders.

12.3.1 Autism

A neurodevelopmental disorder (also termed pervasive developmental disorder) that is characterized by:

- Difficulties in **social** interactions and **communication**.
- Restricted, **repetitive** interests and patterns of behaviour.
- Onset in **early childhood** (before 36 months) (see Table 12.1).

Impairment varies—spectrum of severity. Autism is usually **identified by 5 years** of age. Subtle, milder deficits may not be identified until later. 'Asperger's

Table 12.1 Clinical features of autism

Social interaction	Communication	Restricted, repetitive behaviours
Abnormal use of eye contact, facial expression, body posture/gesture	Speech delayed, or never develops	Fixation on limited range of interests
Difficulty/disinterest in forming relationships	Failure of normal 'back-and-forth' conversation	Strong preference for routine, distress if routines changed
Lack of 'socio-emotional reciprocity' (response to other people's emotions, understanding social cues)	Unusual patterns of speech, use of 'stock phrase' or accents	Repetitive mannerisms such as hand-flapping, rocking
Lack of seeking to share enjoyment/interests with others	Little imaginative play	Preoccupation with unusual aspects of objects (e.g. the smell or feel of a toy)

syndrome' (ICD-10) is subsumed under the broader heading of autism spectrum disorders (ASD) in DSM-5.

12.3.1.1 Autism: demographics and aetiology

- Male:female 4:1 (more marked gender difference in milder cases).
- Highly heritable, complex, multiple genes (associated with neural connectivity), gene–environment interaction.
- Brain-imaging demonstrates abnormal brain structure, connectivity.
- Not caused by MMR vaccine or cold/indifferent mothering style (common myths).

12.3.1.2 Autism: clinical presentation

For a diagnosis of autism, clinical features (see Table 12.1) must be **pervasive** (present in all situations) and, reflecting the neurodevelopmental underpinning of this disorder, present before age 3 years.

12.3.1.3 Autism: treatment

There is no specific treatment. Interventions are focused on:

- Optimizing the individual's potential.
- Identifying and treating co-morbidities.
- Early recognition.

Interventions include psycho-education, behavioural modification techniques, and optimization of educational setting.

Medications do not benefit core deficits of autism. They should be used with caution and only if other, less invasive, interventions are ineffective. **Start with a low dose** and **slowly titrate** according to response and tolerability. Examples include:

- Behavioural problems: atypical antipsychotic may help with aggression (risperidone, aripiprazole).
- ADHD (see Section 12.3.4) but note risk of sensitivity to side-effects.
- Anxiety/depression: SSRIs (also used in self-injurious behaviour).
- Initial insomnia: melatonin.

12.3.2 Asperger's syndrome

- Classified separately within pervasive development disorders (PDDs) (ICD 10) but subsumed within ASD (DSM-5).
- Commonalities with autism include (milder) social and communication difficulties, and restricted patterns of interest; difficulties in reading

non-verbal/social cues, social 'awkwardness', overly formal approach to others, and unusual patterns of speech.

- Unlike autism, usually no speech or cognitive delay.
- Often diagnosed much later than autism with early difficulties only recognized retrospectively.
- Undiagnosed, individuals may develop anxiety/depression due to difficulties in social settings.

12.3.3 Rett's syndrome

- Least common example of PDD.
- X-linked (sporadic mutations of the MECP2 gene on X chromosome).
- Occurs in girls.
- Onset before 2 years.
- 'Normal' early development followed by gradual loss of speech and motor skills.
- Prominent 'hand-wringing movements'.
- Severe learning disability (usually).

12.3.4 Attention deficit hyperactivity disorder (ADHD)
Common neurodevelopmental disorder.

12.3.4.1 ADHD: clinical presentation
See Table 12.2.
Symptoms:

- Present in at least two settings (e.g. home and school).
- From an early age (before 6years for ICD 10).

Table 12.2 ADHD clinical triad

Inattention	Hyperactivity	Impulsivity
• Careless mistakes in schoolwork	• Fidgety/restless	• Talks excessively
• Difficulty sustaining attention	• Leaves seat in classroom	• Blurts out answers
• Appears not to listen	• Always on the go ('as if driven by a motor')	• Difficulty waiting turn
• Doesn' complete instructions/tasks	• Climbs/runs excessively	• Intrusive with others
• Forgetful/distractible	• Difficulty with quiet play	
• Disorganized/frequently loses things		

- Cause significant functional impairment.
- In all three domains (ICD-10), inattention or hyperactivity or both (DSM-5).

Co-morbid disorders (up to 50%):

- Oppositional defiant/conduct.
- Autism spectrum.
- Anxiety/depression.
- Substance abuse.

12.3.4.2 ADHD: demographics and aetiology

- Prevalence: 1–2% (ICD 10), 3–5% (DSM-5)—higher in areas of social deprivation.
- Male:female = 3–4:1.
- Highly heritable—multiple 'risk-genes', role in dopamine function and neuronal development, main theories relate to catecholamine dysfunction.
- Environmental risks include obstetric complications (prematurity/low birth-weight, prenatal exposure to alcohol, nicotine, and benzodiazepines), gene–environment interactions important.
- Brain—abnormalities in frontal, temporal cortices, basal ganglia, cerebellum. Longitudinal brain-imaging suggests possible neural maturation delay. Normalization of brain structure correlates with reduction in ADHD symptoms.

12.3.4.3 ADHD: management

Untreated, the inattention, hyperactivity and impulsivity associated with ADHD lead to increased risk of substance misuse, co-morbid mental illness, and criminal behaviour. Effectively treated, this risk can be significantly reduced. The **goals of treatment** are to:

- Ensure that the child **reaches their potential**, educationally and socially.
- **Reduce distress**, for the child and their social circle.

12.3.4.3.1 Non-pharmacological interventions

Support the relationship between the child and their parents/teachers, promoting a **consistent** approach to communication, rule-setting, and co-ordination between care-givers. **Reinforcement** of positive behaviours and appropriate consequences for problem behaviours, social skills training, and CBT. While non-pharmacological approaches reduce oppositionality and improve the parent–child relationship, they have limited effectiveness in treating core features of moderate/severe disorder.

12.3.4.3.2 Pharmacological interventions

Medication, due to significant side-effects, reserved for those with moderate-severe symptomatology (NICE guidelines), includes stimulants and non-stimulants.

12.3.4.3.3 Stimulants

- Reduce hyperactivity, mechanism unknown (monoamine transporter inhibitors—noradrenaline and dopamine).
- **Methylphenidate** (short- and long-acting), **lisdexamfetamine** (second-line).
- Start with short-acting forms (about 4 h) to assess efficacy/tolerability. If respond, switch to long-acting to provide symptom-control for 8–12 h. Reduces hyperactivity, impulsivity, improves attention.
- 'Drug holidays' (medication not administered for periods) only if marked side-effects (e.g. anorexia causing weight loss).
- Children re-assessed off medication (generally annually) to assess for spontaneous remission and need for medication, as the disorder improves with age.
- If medication helpful, children may need to use it for years (some parents reluctant).
- **Monitoring** is essential:
  - o Weight, height on **centile charts** (appetite and weight loss).
  - o Physical examination pre-treatment (identify cardiac abnormalities).
  - o ECG may be necessary, BP and HR monitored regularly.
  - o Response (ADHD rating-scales completed by parents and schools).
  - o Side-effects and adherence.

12.3.4.3.4 Non-stimulants

- Generally used if stimulants are unhelpful/intolerable.
- **Atomoxetine** blocks noradrenaline re-uptake (in contrast to stimulants takes up to 12 weeks to have full effect).
- **Guanfacine**, selective alpha-2a receptor agonist, may be useful for oppositionality associated with ADHD, often given with stimulants in USA (not yet licensed everywhere).
- As with stimulants, HR and BP should be monitored.

12.3.4.4 ADHD: prognosis

ADHD can persist (up to 60%) into adulthood with psychiatric co-morbidity, social, and occupational impairment.

12.3.5 Tic disorders

Vocal/motor tics (repetitive, stereotyped actions) are common, often transient, in school-age children. They may be simple (brief, meaningless, e.g. blinking) or complex (more purposeful movements, e.g. jumping). **Tourette's syndrome** presents with frequent complex motor (and vocal) tics. Pre-pubertal onset of tics and/ or OCD, associated with group A beta-haemolytic streptococcal infection, constitute a group of paediatric autoimmune neuropsychiatric disorders (**PANDAs**) believed to have an autoimmune aetiology. Generally, tics are transient, improving with age. Poorer prognosis is associated with Tourette's and OCD.

12.4 Oppositional defiant disorder (ODD)/conduct disorder (CD)

These separate disorders are described together due to similar aetiologies and presentations. Core features include **persistent, severe:**

- Disobedience.
- Defiance.
- Hostility.
- **Conduct disorder** also includes aggressive, **antisocial problem-behaviours** (associated with later dissocial personality disorder).

Problem-behaviours:
- Physical aggression toward siblings.
- Temper tantrums.
- Later childhood:
  ○ Persistent stealing.
  ○ Lying.
  ○ Verbal and physical aggression.
- With **older age,** problems outside the home become more evident:
  ○ Truancy.
  ○ Vandalism.
  ○ Substance abuse.
  ○ Promiscuity.
  ○ Fire setting (rare).

ICD-10 requires at least three symptoms (from list of 15), persisting over time (minimum 6 months)—distinguishes transient response to environmental stressor.

12.4.1 ODD/CD: demographics and aetiology
- Prevalence rates vary—1 to 6% (higher in lower socioeconomic groups).
- Male:female = 2:1.
- Cause unclear, environmental factors important, genetic factors may contribute via effect on temperament.

- Risk factors include:
  - o Low socio-economic status.
  - o Parental mental illness/substance use/criminality.
  - o Abuse/neglect.
- Antenatal exposure to toxins, e.g. nicotine, lead.

12.4.2 ODD/CD: management

- Depends on severity.
- **Parental support programmes** (NICE) for younger children (12 years and under): identifying inadvertent reinforcement of problem-behaviours, re-inforcing positive-behaviours.
- Treat **co-morbidities** (e.g. ADHD, depression).
- Medication occasionally used (psychological interventions unsuccessful), e.g. severe aggression (atypical antipsychotic).

See Practical tips Interventions in children.

12.4.3 ODD/CD: prognosis

- Varies.
- Poorer prognosis:
  - o Severe.
  - o Early onset.
  - o Parental mental illness, criminality.

Practical tips Interventions in children

Most interventions focus on psychological strategies, delivered by MDT, including:
- Assessment of child/parent interactions and environment.
- Identify stressors, parental conflict/inconsistencies, inadvertent reinforcement of challenging behaviour.
- Interventions to address these, including reducing stressors (where possible), educating and supporting parents, support for children.

12.5 Anxiety disorders

This section will focus on **presentations specific to childhood**: separation anxiety disorder, school refusal, and selective mutism. Anxiety is part of normal experience. Children experience fears that may be age-appropriate, including fear of strangers, the dark, social situations. It is severity, pervasive-ness, and functional impairment that define the disorders that follow. As with all presentations, careful assessment is essential (see Clinical vignette Child-psychiatry assessment).

12.5.1 Separation anxiety disorder

- Intense fear of separation from a person to whom the child is attached, fears harm will befall them, they will leave them.
- Persists beyond toddler years and/or significantly impairs function.
- Refuse to be apart from attachment figure, experience physical symptoms of anxiety.
- May be precipitated by a single experience or prolonged difficulties (e.g. parental conflict), or over-protective parenting.
- More common in girls.
- Often co-morbid with other anxiety disorders.

12.5.1.1 Separation anxiety disorder: treatment

- Psychological interventions—reduction of stressors, focus on parents' approach.
- Short-term medication (not the mainstay of treatment) in **severe** cases (e.g. cannot engage in psychological interventions) (expert guidance).

Clinical vignette Child-psychiatry assessment

'I had recently started as a child-psychiatry trainee in a major London-teaching hospital. I assessed my first patient—an 8-year old boy with intense anxiety, fear of the dark, separation anxiety, and evolving school refusal. Accompanied by his mother, he seemed to engage well. His mother gave very little information. I devised a behavioural intervention, including graded return to school, support for his mother, and the purchase of a night-light for his room. I did not do a home-visit, nor did I have any knowledge of where he lived in inner-city London. At review 2 weeks later, he was worse, distressed and tearful. Collateral history from his mother revealed that their family dog had been killed (throat slit and left on their door-step) and a rock thrown through the child's bedroom window had smashed both the window and the night-light.

'That was a sobering experience, and one I have never forgotten. Proper assessment, particularly in children, must include full knowledge of the child's environment and supports.' Consultant Psychiatrist

---

12.5.3 School refusal

- Not distinct disorder, usually a presentation of an underlying disorder such as separation anxiety, social anxiety disorder, depression, or a specific phobia relating to aspects of school life such as public transport.

- Distinguish from **truancy** (child chooses not to go to school) or child being kept at home.
- Increasing reluctance to go to school with frequent somatic complaints (not present on non-school days) when time for school, eventually refuses altogether.
- Majority eventually return, some do not and social problems may persist.

12.5.3.1 *School refusal: treatment*

- Treat underlying issues, get child back to school as soon as possible.
- Liaise with the school; may be helpful for someone other than the parent to accompany the child to school. Graded re-introduction to school, training in anxiety-management strategies.
- Change of school may be necessary.

12.5.4 Selective mutism

- Speaks normally in some situations but not others (e.g. normal at home, mutism in school).
- Usually no inherent abnormality of speech, language.
- Co-morbid anxiety disorder.
- Onset generally 3–5 years.
- Assessment difficult given child's refusal to speak. History reliant on parents' collateral. It is important to clarify that speech and comprehension are normal at home. Relevant differential diagnoses, such as PDDs, should be excluded before a diagnosis is made.
- Treatment usually behavioural with positive reinforcement but problems often persist with long-term social difficulties.

12.6 **Mood disorders**

Criteria for mood disorders in childhood are the same as for adults (see Chapter 6). Sections 12.6.1 and 12.6.2 illustrate points **particularly relevant for children/ adolescents.**

12.6.1 Depression

- Low mood may not be as prominent.
- Behaviour (social withdrawal, academic decline) may be presenting signs (may also represent early psychosis).
- Somatic symptoms more common, particularly in younger children who cannot identify emotions.
- Do not dismiss as 'normal' adolescent difficulties.

12.6.1.1 Depression: management

- Psychological interventions: CBT, family therapy.
- Moderate-severe depression may need medication. Start low, 'go slow', often starting with 1/8 of the dose you expect to reach (e.g. 2.5 mg fluoxetine daily). Monitor carefully—higher risks of suicidal thoughts/impulsivity. Seek expert advice.

12.6.2 Bipolar disorder

- Concern about appropriateness of adult criteria: behaviour considered disinhibited, grandiose in an adult may be normal for the developmental stage of the child; possible overlap with other childhood disorders (e.g. ADHD).
- Diagnosis of BPAD necessitates the prescribing of medication with potentially serious adverse effects (e.g. lithium)—careful assessment needed. Conversely, must not deny treatment to an ill adolescent.
- Other diagnoses (PDD, psychotic disorders, substance abuse, or organic causes) must be excluded.

12.6.2.1 Bipolar disorder: management

- Prescribing based on data from adults (caution).
- Atypical antipsychotics (risperidone/aripiprazole) and sodium valproate to stabilize mood. Evidence that lithium is not as effective if started and then stopped, so, while effective, usually not used at this age.
- Psychological support for families and patients.

12.7 Psychotic disorders in childhood/adolescence

Criteria are the same as for adults (see Chapter 7). The following sections illustrate points **particularly relevant for children**.

12.7.1 Psychotic disorders: clinical presentation

- Psychotic **symptoms** not uncommon in childhood, a diagnosis of schizophrenia is rare, although adolescence does not preclude a diagnosis.
- Gradual change in social, academic functioning, pre-dating overt psychotic symptoms, termed '**prodrome**', may be missed or mistaken for depression.
- More likely to present with **disorganized** thought/behaviour, negative symptoms, rather than delusions/hallucinations.
- More common in males.
- Important to exclude substance abuse, PDD, or organic illnesses, e.g. epilepsy.

12.7.2 Psychotic disorders: management

- Long duration of untreated psychosis associated with poorer outcome—early intervention to identify high-risk individuals key.
- Challenging—not everyone who displays prodromal symptoms will go on to develop psychotic symptoms—difficult to justify antipsychotics in someone who is not, and may never be, psychotic.
- Literature on **antipsychotics** largely based on adults:
  O Risperidone licensed for use for children aged 5–18 years with persistent aggression in conduct disorder.
  O Adolescents particularly sensitive to adverse effects (e.g. EPSEs)—caution.
  O Growing recognition of significant risk of cardio-metabolic complications.
- **Psychological interventions** (problem-solving, social skills training, family therapy) helpful in non-acute phase.

12.7.3 Psychotic disorders: prognosis

- Poor prognosis.
- Disruption to normal psychosocial development.
- Increased cognitive deficits, negative symptoms.

12.8 Perinatal mental illness

- Women are at greater risk of developing mental illness during the perinatal period than at any other time (relapse of established illness or first presentation).
- Pro-active management important due to potential **impact of maternal mental illness,** including:
  O Failure to engage with **antenatal care** (poorer obstetric outcomes—low birth-weight (LBW), prematurity).
  O Impact of substance abuse.
  O Disturbance of mother–baby bonding (associated with childhood difficulties).
  O Direct risk to baby:
    - **Neglect**—unable for basic (feeding, washing, etc.) or emotional needs.
    - **Rarely**—thoughts of harming the child—may be obsessional/anxious.

12.8.1 Assessment before/during pregnancy

- Ask all pregnant women about **personal, family psychiatric history** (including post-partum psychosis).
- Medication should generally be **avoided.**
- For women with **severe mental illness,** medication may be continued if benefits outweigh risks—seek specialist advice.

- Decisions should be made on a case-by-case basis considering:
  - Diagnosis, consequences of previous relapses, current and previous treatments, mother's preference.
  - **General advice** if using medications in pregnancy—use:
    - Minimum effective dose.
    - Monotherapy where possible.
  - Some agents are **never** used, e.g. sodium valproate (anti-epileptic and mood stabilizer) due to high risk of teratogenicity.
  - In **major disorders**, particularly BPAD, discuss (and document) **pregnancy planning**, risk of relapse (increased eight-fold postnatally in BPAD), and risk/benefit of treatment. Discussion should include:
    - Identification of their early signs of relapse.
    - Designation of another person (e.g. partner) who can monitor and contact services, if concerned.

12.8.2 Specific psychotropics in pregnancy

Seek specialist advice if unclear and consult up-to-date guidelines (e.g. British National Formulary (BNF)).

12.8.2.1 SSRIs

SSRIs are associated with several complications:

- Low birth-weight, pre-term delivery (depression may be a confounding factor).
- **Neonatal adaptation syndrome** (NAS)—assumed to be a form of withdrawal, varies in severity.
- Infant is 'jittery', has difficulties feeding.
- Self-limiting.
- More marked with medications with a short half-life.
- Persistent **pulmonary hypertension** in the neonate (evidence limited, increase in risk is small).
- **Sertraline** is considered to be one of the safer anti-depressants to use in pregnancy and breastfeeding. Although all anti-depressants are excreted in breast milk, sertraline is present in lower quantities compared to other anti-depressants.
- **Fluoxetine** has been in use for some time and, therefore, more experience with its use in pregnancy.
- **Paroxetine** is associated with an increased risk of cardiovascular malformations and is **best avoided** in pregnancy.
- There is **little information** about newer agents, e.g. venlafaxine.

12.8.2.2 Antipsychotics

- Evidence for safety in pregnancy limited; however, psychoses are themselves associated with adverse outcomes (pre-term delivery, low birthweights, congenital anomalies).
- Consider carefully any decision to stop antipsychotics in pregnancy—the risk of relapse is high.
- First-generation antipsychotics (e.g. chlorpromazine) may be preferred as there is more experience with their use in pregnancy.
- **Atypical antipsychotics are not considered safer in pregnancy** (increased risk metabolic complications, e.g. gestational diabetes). Olanzapine is probably most commonly used. Less evidence for novel agents (e.g. aripiprazole).
- **Clozapine** in pregnancy is uncommon but risk of relapse for those stable on clozapine is significant—seek specialist advice. Breastfeeding is contraindicated. Given the increase in total blood volume and GFR during pregnancy, blood levels of clozapine will drop during the 3rd trimester and an increase in dose may be necessary. The dose must be adjusted post-delivery—monitor levels.

12.8.2.3 Mood stabilizers

- Women with BPAD are at particular risk of relapse during pregnancy, especially post-partum. For this reason, a **clear plan** should be in place.
- If there is a plan to withdraw medication, withdraw gradually pre-conception.
- Women and their partners should be informed that many relapse perinatally.
- **Lithium** is associated with cardiac malformation (Ebstein's anomaly). Actual risk is small (1:2000) and must be balanced with risk of relapse. Many women continue lithium during pregnancy. If they experience significant nausea/vomiting, they may develop **lithium toxicity**. As with clozapine, haemo-dilution in the 3rd trimester may necessitate dose increase, with reduction to pre-pregnancy doses after delivery. Lithium is held at the start of labour and re-commenced after delivery. Monitor levels and renal profile closely.
- **Sodium valproate** is **contra-indicated** in women of child-bearing age (increased risk of neural tube defects). It is also linked with cardiac malformations.
- **Carbamazepine** and **lamotrigine** are also associated with an increased risk of neural tube defects. Lamotrigine is associated with an increased risk of cleft palate.
- **Note:** taking folic acid prior to conception does not remove the risk of neural tube defects secondary to anti-epileptics/mood stabilizers.

12.8.3 Loss of foetus and still-birth

- May be associated with significant distress.
- Support and monitor for depression.

12.9 Disorders of the postnatal period

12.9.1 Baby blues (postnatal blues)

- **NOT** a mental illness.
- Common.
- Transient disturbance of mood/emotions 3–5 days post-delivery.
- Typical features:
  - Tearfulness.
  - Irritability/lability.
  - Insomnia.
  - More common in first time mothers.
  - Possible hormonal aetiology.
- Self-limiting—usually resolves within a week.
- Persistent symptoms may be risk factor for postnatal depression.

12.9.2 Postnatal depression (PND)

- Usually within first 2–3 months.
- **10-15%** of women.
- **Risk** factors:
  - Personal/family history of depression.
  - Limited support system.
  - Poor self-esteem.
  - Obstetric complications.

12.9.2.1 PND: clinical features

- May be dismissed as 'normal'—important not to miss more profound difficulties.
- Usual symptoms of depression but often focus on baby:
  - **Worry** about baby's health/well-being.
  - **Guilt** about impact of symptoms on baby.
  - **Doubt** about their abilities as a mother.
  - **Guilt** they aren't enjoying motherhood more.
  - **Anxiety** may be prominent.
- If severe, may be unable to appropriately care for their baby.

Note: It is **normal** for new parents to worry—it is the **persistence** and **prominence** of these worries, the presence of other **depressive** symptoms, and their **functional impact** that suggests depression.

12.9.2.2 PND: assessment

As with depression but with **additional assessment of risk for the baby.** Questions should be asked in a compassionate, non-judgemental way, but must include:

- Ability to care for the baby.
- Thoughts of harm to self or baby.
- Past history of harm to self or others.
- Psychotic symptoms, especially pertaining to the baby.
- Active substance use.
- Clarifying available supports.

(Knowledge of local child protection procedures is necessary should you need child welfare services.) If concerned about safety, admission may be necessary.

12.9.2.3 PND: management

Treatment is the same as at any other stage but with the additional impact of **breastfeeding** and **a small baby** (both its safety and stress for the mother):

- **Mild** depression **psychological intervention**, improving supports, regular review.
- **Moderate-severe** depression—anti-depressants, CBT.
- If breastfeeding, avoid drugs if possible (many excreted in breast milk).

12.9.3 Post-partum psychosis

This is a **psychiatric emergency**. The majority are **affective psychoses** occurring in women with underlying mood disorder (usually BPAD). Occasionally, it is a first presentation:

- 90% present within 2 weeks of delivery, peak onset in first 48 h.
- Risk is significantly higher with a history of BPAD, family or personal history of post-partum psychosis (up to 80-90% if manic relapse).

12.9.3.1 Post-partum psychosis: clinical presentation

- Mix of mood (mainly manic) and psychotic symptoms, fluctuate rapidly.
- Features include:
  o Perplexity.
  o Agitation.

○ Insomnia.

○ Psychotic symptoms (may be 'first-rank').

12.9.3.2 Post-partum psychosis: assessment

- Rule out organic cause, e.g. delirium.
- Assess psychotic symptoms carefully to identify if they pertain to baby.
- Careful risk assessment-incorporating risk to mother and to the baby.

12.9.3.3 Post-partum psychosis: management

- Very unlikely to be able to care for baby. Ideally, both admitted to a mother-and-baby unit.
- Acute phase—antipsychotics plus anxiolytic/hypnotic, as required.
- Other medications (anti-depressants, mood stabilizers) depend on underlying diagnosis.
- May not be appropriate/able to breastfeed.
- ECT may be considered in this setting (rapid response).
- Psycho-education (including family).
- Women should be closely monitored, including assessment of the mother–baby bond.
- A diagnosis of post-partum psychosis has **significant implications for future** pregnancies. Women (and their partners) should be made aware of risks and given clear advice and support.

12.10 Summary

Each stage of childhood may present with mental illness. These have many characteristics of adult mental illness, but several either have particular features or are specific to the developmental stage. Psycho-social interventions, provided by a well-functioning MDT, are key in all mental illness, but particularly in this group. The complexities of prescribing medication for them means that, if medications are required, you are likely to need expert advice.

CHAPTER 13

Psychiatry of intellectual disability (ID)

<table>
<tr><td>CHAPTER FOCUS</td></tr>
</table>

What you should know about the psychiatry of intellectual disability (ID)

- What is meant by ID
- Causes and comorbidities of ID.
- What impact ID may have on the presentation of mental and physical illness.
- How to manage challenging behaviours.
- Specific issues in assessing and managing ID.

13.1 Introduction

This chapter discusses the mental health needs of people with intellectual disability (ID). The terms used to describe intellectual (learning) disability vary, as some have gained pejorative associations. 'Intellectual disability' is still used, but this may change with ICD-11 and the introduction of the term intellectual developmental disorders (IDD)—a concept of neuro-developmental disorders with global impairment in general intellectual functioning, including planning, judgement, learning, and abstract thinking. People with ID present with physical and mental illness and it is important to be aware of the impact of ID on these presentations (see Clinical vignette Presentation of ID in the ED).

> ### Clinical vignette—Presentation of ID in the ED
>
> 'I was the psychiatry SHO on-call for ED when I was called to assess a 28-year-old single lady with a known diagnosis of mild ID and Down's syndrome, accompanied by her carers. She had lived at a care home for the previous 8 years and was very settled. However, her behaviour had become increasingly bizarre over the previous 3 weeks. She was very over-active, constantly pacing through the house, speaking rapidly, flitting from topic to topic. She had also become very disinhibited, making sexual advances to the carers, and dressing inappropriately. She was awake for most of the night over the previous 10 days and wanted to leave most evenings—something she had never done previously. Her carers were very upset, finding it increasingly difficult to manage her. One of the residents had died 4 weeks previously and they felt this had had a huge impact on the patient. Her key worker had moved to a different residence 3 months previously.
>
> *continued >*

> 'She was extremely agitated and distressed, dishevelled, shouting, and very in-appropriate in her interaction with other patients. She appeared breathless and a little cyanosed. I did not know where to start... Even though I work as a GP now, I have never forgotten the complexity of that presentation'. GP

13.2 Definitions and levels of severity in ID

Current WHO (ICD-10) guidelines define intellectual disability ('mental retard-ation') as a 'condition of arrested or incomplete development of the mind' characterized by:

- Significant global impairment of intelligence.
- Significant impairment of social or adaptive functioning that arose during the developmental period.

An alternative definition, proposed by the Department of Health (Ireland), is 'a significantly reduced ability to:

- understand new or complex information;
- learn new skills (impaired intelligence);
- cope independently (impaired social functioning);

starting before adulthood, with a lasting effect on development'.

The WHO defines **disabilities** as an umbrella term covering:

- **Impairment**: abnormality of structure or function (e.g. impairment in brain function with respect to visual and auditory information processing).
- **Activity limitation**: reduction of ability to perform due to impairment (severe dyslexia secondary to the above).
- **Participation restriction**: a disadvantage for a given person that limits or prevents their role fulfilment (e.g. unable to pass school tests despite normal intelligence as they require reading—this may be overcome if other strategies, e.g. audiobooks, taping lectures, etc. are used). It is important to consider the part society plays in restricting an individual's participation.

Intelligence can be considered as the sum of those cognitive abilities (e.g. reasoning, planning, critical thinking, creativity, etc.) that underline **adaptation to one's environment**. It is assessed using intelligence tests and the results are often reported as intelligence quotient (IQ). In children, this is calculated by:

$$IQ = \frac{\text{Mental Age}}{\text{Chronological Age}} \times 100$$

Table 13.1 Severity and clinical picture in ID				
Severity of ID	IQ range	Mental age (years)	Prevalence	Clinical picture (ICD 10)
Mild	50-69	9-12	2.5%	**Language** acquisition delayed but can use speech for everyday purposes—frequent reading and writing problems **Self-care** mostly independent **Tasks**—capable of practical tasks **Social and emotional** immaturity
Moderate	35-49	6-9	0.4%	**Language** acquisition slow, eventual achievement limited **Self-care**—support required **Tasks**—simple practical work under supervision
Severe	20-34	3-6	0.1%	**Language** acquisition very limited, relies on gestures, facial expression and photographs or objects to communicate **Self-care**—significant support required **Tasks**—support required for daily routines
Profound	<20	<3		**Language** limited to simple commands/ requests. Often non-verbal **Self-care**—24-h care and supervision **Tasks**—can learn some new skills but very slowly Multiple **physical disabilities** common

The severity of intellectual disability, defined by IQ, is reflected in the clinical picture (see Table 13.1)

13.3 Aetiology of ID

As with mental illness, in many cases of mild learning disability (and some more severe cases), the aetiology is likely to be an interaction between genetic predisposition (linked to multiple, small genetic contributions) and environmental

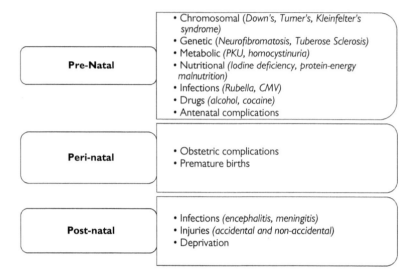

Pre-Natal
- Chromosomal (*Down's, Turner's, Kleinfelter's syndrome*)
- Genetic (*Neurofibromatosis, Tuberose Sclerosis*)
- Metabolic (*PKU, homocystinuria*)
- Nutritional (*Iodine deficiency, protein-energy malnutrition*)
- Infections (*Rubella, CMV*)
- Drugs (*alcohol, cocaine*)
- Antenatal complications

Peri-natal
- Obstetric complications
- Premature births

Post-natal
- Infections (*encephalitis, meningitis*)
- Injuries (*accidental and non-accidental*)
- Deprivation

Figure 13.1 Specific causes of intellectual disability.

factors. Identification of underlying aetiology (Figure 13.1), if possible, is important as it informs:

- Prognosis.
- Interventions.
- Advice for parents on future risk.

Some disorders are associated with specific behaviours ('behavioural phenotypes'), e.g. Lesch–Nyhan syndrome and self-harm.

13.4 Co-morbidities in ID

Co-morbidities are common in ID, often correlating with severity. They influence presentation and must be identified and managed. (See Practical tips Key features in learning disability.)

- Physical:
  - Epilepsy (mild ID 4%, moderate/severe ID 30%, severe ID 50%).
  - Motor disabilities (e.g. spasticity, ataxia).
  - Sensory impairment (hearing, vision).

- Mental:
  - Can present as **disordered behaviour** (aggression, self-injury, withdrawal, and stereotypies). A **change** in **behaviour** or level of functioning in someone with an ID must be **investigated**. Presentation can be **wrongly attributed to ID** ('diagnostic over-shadowing').

Practical tips Key features in learning disability

Be aware of co-morbid physical illness (epilepsy, motor disability, e.g. spasticity, ataxia).
Recent deterioration in function or behaviour consider:

- Mental illness.
- Stressful life event/environment.
- Epilepsy (recent onset).
- Other physical causes, e.g. infection.
- Frustration due to lack of communication/sensory impairment.
- Side-effects of medication.

13.5 Challenging behaviours in ID

Some persons with ID present with 'challenging behaviours'. This is not a diagnosis. It simply states that the person's behaviour is deemed challenging by others, presenting risk to the physical safety of the person or others, or likely to result in the person being unable to access facilities. It may serve a function for the person (e.g. communicating distress or avoiding demands). Behaviours defined as challenging include:

- Anti-social behaviour.
- Self-injury, e.g. head-banging.
- Stereotyped behaviours, e.g. rocking, flapping (may lead to misdiagnosis of autism).
- Hyperactivity.

Managing these behaviours requires:

- Careful **assessment** to identify underlying factors (in the person or the environment), e.g.
  - Physical health (e.g. epilepsy).
  - Mental health (e.g. psychosis).
  - Psycho-social issues (e.g. bereavement, carer stress).

Table 13.2 Strategies for the management of challenging behaviours in ID

Proactive (prevent the behaviour)	Reactive (immediate when behaviour occurs)
Reducing factors that increase the likelihood of the behaviour (medical factors, sensory impairments)	Low arousal approaches (e.g. soft, minimal speech, appropriate stance, reduction in stimulation)
Teaching skills to improve wellbeing and tolerance (communication, coping strategies, social networks etc.)	Making the environment safe Providing immediate support

- Robust interventions that respond to specific factors identified and include both proactive and reactive strategies (see Table 13.2).

13.6 Mental illness in ID

13.6.1 Clinical features of mental illness in the context of ID

Mental health problems are common in ID and are influenced by the presence of the ID (see Table 13.3).

13.6.2 Aetiology of mental illness in ID

As with mental illness generally, the underlying aetiology is likely to be multi-factorial. However, factors associated with the underlying ID must be considered.

13.6.2.1 Biological

- Brain pathology (epilepsy, congenital disorders).
- Specific abnormalities (Prader–Willi, fragile X, Lesch–Nyhan).
- Family history of mental illness or learning disability/other brain disorders.
- Iatrogenic.
- Communication and sensory impairments.

13.6.2.2 Psychological

- Childhood experiences.
- Separation, rejection, overprotection, abuse.
- Poor personality development (low self-esteem, dependency, low expectations).
- Life events (bereavement, difficulties making and maintaining relationships, institutionalization, labelling).
- Societal reactions (stigma, isolation, poor support, abuse).

Table 13.3 Epidemiology and characteristics of mental illness in individuals with ID

Mental Disorder	Epidemiology	Characteristics
Prolonged bereavement reactions	Common	Carers are often unaware. Problems may be attributed to other causes. May manifest months after the bereavement.
Depression	Depression and anxiety are up to four times more common in individuals with ID compared to the general population Associated with Down's syndrome	Often missed as individuals with ID are less likely to complain of depressed mood. Biological symptoms are important
Bipolar affective disorder	Estimated prevalence between 0.9-4.8%	Can be diagnosed whatever the degree of disability In manic states irritability is common Recording behavioural correlates of mood can help to establish the cyclical nature, and to monitor treatment
Schizophrenia	Prevalence of 3%	Difficult to diagnose in individuals with IQ <45 Psychotic phenomena tend to be simpler, thought alienation less Bizarre behaviour and adaptive regression can occur
Acute confusional state (delirium)	More common especially in individuals with severe ID or coexistent dementia	Due to physical illness—will need careful diagnosis and treatment
Dementia	Strong association with Down's syndrome (early presentation)	Psychotic symptoms and epilepsy may be features
Autism	Prevalence of 18.4%	To diagnose, symptoms must be present in early childhood but may not become fully manifest until social demands exceed capacities

13.6.2.3 *Social*

- Limited occupational choice.
- Social isolation and limited peer relationships
- Lack of role models in developing adaptive skills.

13.7 Assessment in ID

As communication may be limited, careful and thorough assessment is essential, with **collateral** information from multiple sources.
  Consider:

- **Diagnostic over-shadowing**—tendency to ascribe everything to the ID.
- Baseline exaggeration.
- Physical co-morbidities.

Understand:

- Recent life-events.
- Level of support.
- Daily living skills and activities.
- Role of carers.

Carry out **observations** noting:

- Dysmorphic features.
- Abnormal **movements.**
- Poor self-care.

Assess:

- **Mood** via **associated phenomena**, such as level of interest, engagement, energy, and sleep.
- Consider use of diagnostic or screening **tools** as adjunct to the assessment (e.g. psychiatric assessment schedule—adults with developmental disability, Nisonger child behaviour rating form).
- **Risk** to:
  o Self and others.
  o Exploitation, abuse.

Investigate:

- Bloods—screen for physical illness.
- Additional investigations, e.g. EEG if epilepsy suspected.
- Collateral and reports—for underlying cause of ID if defined.

Practical tips The 7 'C's of assessment in ID

- Be **calm**—allow extra time.
- Be **clear**—ask simple questions.
- Be **creative**—use non-verbal, as well as verbal, communication (gestures, facial expression).
- Be **conscious**—of potential sensory impairment (hearing, vision) and other physical problems.
- Be **competent**—use broad assessments to identify mental illness (e.g. physical manifestations of depression).
- Be **compassionate**—follow the patient's lead for speed and pace.
- Be **collaborative**—always check collateral history, particularly carers, previous reports.

13.8 Management principles in ID

13.8.1 General principles

- Careful assessment (see Practical tips The 7 'C's of assessment in ID).
- Identify **social** and **environmental** issues.
- Assess (and manage):
  - Physical impairments.
  - Communication difficulties.
  - Physical or mental disorder.

The focus is on **normalization**. People with ID should experience normal (or-dinary) lives (where possible, with supports as needed).

A **range of services** should be available:

- Vocational training.
- Day-centres.
- Home and employment support.
- Respite admissions.

The **multi-disciplinary team** is key.

13.8.2 Specific interventions for mental illness

As with any mental illness, management should follow a bio-psycho-social approach.

13.8.2.1 Psycho-social strategies

- Family—education and support (e.g. respite admissions, home-care support).
- Social strategies:
  - ○ Inclusion (community)—dignity, respect, value.
  - ○ Skills' training.
  - ○ Environmental review.
- Behavioural strategies.
- Modified CBT.

13.8.2.2 Biological strategies

The same strategies for mental illness apply to mental illness in an ID setting with some **caveats:**

- Medications are used **sparingly,** due to significantly increased sensitivity to side-effects, 'start low, go slow'.
- Many anti-epileptic drugs, used as mood stabilizers, can cause **agitation.**
- Psychotropic medication is also used in ID in the management of self-injury, violence, and other behaviours. However, as evidence for these interventions is limited, this should **only** be done under **specialist supervision.**

13.9 Summary

Intellectual disability includes a broad range of intellectual ability and impairment. Patients with ID will present to hospital and other medical settings with mental or physical illness. As students, you need to be aware of the impact of ID on communication and presentation, the importance of carers and families, and know how to assess and provide initial management advice for these complex situations, enlisting the help of specialist teams for ongoing care.

CHAPTER 14

Psychological medicine (hospital psychiatry)

CHAPTER FOCUS

What you should know about psychological medicine
- Broad concepts of mental health in physical settings.
- Effects of medical illness/treatments on mood and well-being.
- Somatoform disorders.
- Neuro-psychiatry—mental health features of epilepsy, stroke, and other neurological disorders.

14.1 Introduction

As one of the authors of this handbook is a liaison psychiatrist, it could be argued that a liaison perspective permeates much of this book. As most doctors will encounter psychiatry in a (non-psychiatric) hospital or medical setting, it could equally be argued that this perspective is most useful in the context of training medical staff. Certainly, many of the topics normally considered under this heading are presented in other chapters. This chapter will, therefore, examine the broad role of liaison psychiatry in medical settings before focusing on some specific areas: neuro-psychiatry, disorders presenting with physical symptoms, and those associated with medical/surgical treatments.

14.2 What is liaison psychiatry and what does it provide?

Psychological medicine (hospital or liaison psychiatry) refers to the interface between medicine and psychiatry—a complex interrelationship (Figure 14.1). It is typically based in a general hospital setting.

In its broadest remit, the liaison psychiatrist provides education, support, and guidance to medical/surgical colleagues, unfamiliar with mental illness, treating patients with co-morbid mental illness (see Clinical vignette Mental illness and medical treatment).

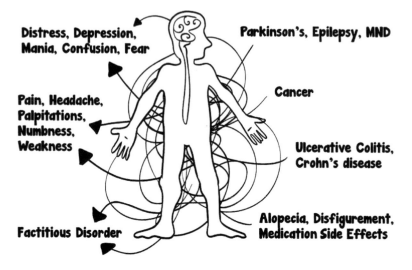

Distress, Depression, Mania, Confusion, Fear

Parkinson's, Epilepsy, MND

Pain, Headache, Palpitations, Numbness, Weakness

Cancer

Ulcerative Colitis, Crohn's disease

Factitious Disorder

Alopecia, Disfigurement, Medication Side Effects

Figure 14.1 The complex relationship between 'physical' and 'psychological' concepts. © Eoin Kelleher.

Clinical vignette Major mental illness and medical treatment

'A 30-year-old, single mother of three had bipolar affective disorder, alcohol dependence and emotionally unstable personality disorder. With limited support, her mood disorder had been difficult to treat, with several manic episodes and multiple episodes of self-harm.

'A recent diagnosis of advanced lung cancer, requiring complex treatment (biological agents and steroids) would prove challenging. It required consistent, weekly support from a senior member of the liaison psychiatry team [consultant] to co-manage the inevitable complications, made more difficult during the Covid pandemic, when many reviews had to be conducted remotely.

'On one occasion, remote review by the psychiatrist noted that the patient was quiet, withdrawn and "flat" in interaction by phone, the patient describing herself as "low, disinterested, and withdrawn". While this could be explained by "depression", the clinical presentation did not fit, and the psychiatrist was concerned about physical causes. Close working-relationships with the oncology team allowed the patient to be transferred directly for medical assessment that revealed pneumonia, bilateral pulmonary emboli, and significant hypokalaemia.' Liaison Psychiatrist

There are numerous examples like this vignette (mental and medical illness): breast cancer presenting in a patient with learning disability and behavioural challenges; acute appendicitis in a patient with schizophrenia; renal failure in a patient on lithium with bipolar affective disorder; leukaemia in a patient with an eating disorder. A well-established liaison psychiatry service, truly embedded within a general hospital, allows complex medical and surgical treatment of patients with complex co-morbid medical and mental illness.

The service also provides rapid assessment and, where appropriate, intervention, for patients attending the general hospital (in-patients/out-patients/ED). This will include rapid, emergency assessments (see Chapter 18), assessment and advice re management of substance abuse (see Chapter 10), eating disorders (see Chapter 9), personality disorders (see Chapter 5), and intellectual disability (see Chapter 13). Delirium is a common reason for referral (see Chapter 11) and liaison psychiatrists can help in more complex assessments of capacity (see Chapter 15). Understanding psychological morbidity is an invaluable skill for physicians and surgeons working with these patients; transmitting this understanding to our student doctors, is the aim of this handbook.

14.3 Specific areas: introduction

There are some areas that are relatively specific to liaison psychiatry:

- Neuro-psychiatry.
- Disorders presenting with physical symptoms.
- Disorders shaped by medical/surgical illness/treatment.

14.4 Neuro-psychiatry

Neuro-psychiatry is an extensive topic. Any disorder affecting the CNS (e.g. head injury, HIV/AIDS, encephalitis) can lead to co-morbid psychiatric symptoms.
This text focuses on three areas:

- Epilepsy.
- Parkinson's disease.
- Stroke.

14.4.1 Epilepsy
Psychiatric presentations are common in epilepsy. These include:

- Syndromes directly attributed to epilepsy.
- Co-morbidities of epilepsy.
- Medication side-effects.

14.4.1.1 Syndromes directly attributed to epilepsy

Pre-ictal (before the seizure):

- Prodromes (anxiety, insomnia, dysphoria).
- Aura, most common in complex partial seizures (e.g. derealization, autonomic symptoms, olfactory hallucinations), linked to pathology in the temporal lobe.

Ictal (during the seizure):

- Automatisms (stereotyped movements, usually purposeless).
- Bizarre behaviour, sometimes aggressive.

Post-ictal (after the seizure):

- Delirium—may last hours, sometimes days. If prolonged may need to outrule persistent seizures.
- Psychosis (may include grandiose, religious or somatic delusions; visual and auditory hallucinations, a strong affective component).

Inter-ictal (between seizures):

- Brief inter-ictal psychosis typically includes paranoid symptoms and hallucinations. Occurs in the context of well-controlled epilepsy.
- 'Chronic' inter-ictal psychosis may be due to repetitive temporal-lobe seizures. It resembles schizophrenia, distinguished by its:
  o Late onset (10–15 years post epilepsy diagnosis).
  o Better preservation of affect and pre-morbid personality.
  o Visual hallucinations.

Co-morbidities of epilepsy include depression and cognitive deterioration. Disentangling these from the primary diagnosis and medication is difficult. Psychotropic medication-use in epilepsy is difficult as many of the antipsychotics lower the seizure threshold. Close liaison with the neurology team is crucial. Benzodiazepines can be useful both in managing seizures and some of the psychological symptoms (distress and agitation).

14.4.2 Parkinson's disease

Primary Parkinson's disease is a degenerative disorder usually presenting in the 6th decade. It is associated with loss of dopaminergic neurons in the substantia nigra of the basal ganglia leading to imbalance in dopaminergic (DA)/acetylcholinergic (ACH) pathways.

Motor symptoms include:

- Tremor: 'pill-rolling', asymmetric, increased by anxiety, decreased by voluntary movement.
- Rigidity: 'cog-wheel' or 'lead-pipe'.
- Bradykinesia: slowing of movement, elicited by finger tap speed, pronation/supination movements.
- Postural instability.

Non-motor symptoms include:

- Cognitive dysfunction and dementia (independent predictor of mortality).
- Sleep disturbance.
- Fatigue.
- Autonomic dysfunction.
- Pain and sensory disturbance.
- Anxiety, depression.
- Psychosis (usually due to medications, e.g. anticholinergics, levodopa). Because of the complex overlap between the DA-enhancing medications used to treat Parkinson's disease, and side-effects (such as hallucinations and paranoid delusions), treatment can be very difficult. The initial step in managing psychosis in the setting of Parkinson's disease is to try to reduce DA agonists. Addition of quetiapine or clozapine may be necessary. SSRIs may worsen Parkinson's disease symptoms. Pramipexole (a dopamine agonist) is helpful in patients with depression in the context of Parkinson's disease.

14.4.3 Stroke

Stroke may present with a range of issues, including depression, cognitive impairment, emotional lability, and personality change. The presentation is often influenced by the site of the lesion. **Post-stroke depression** (PSD) is common, found in more than a third of cases. Likely contributing factors include the underlying brain injury (left-sided lesions particularly associated with depression) and the psychological impact of the sudden disability. Typically, post-stroke depression differs from major depression (in addition to the presence of a stroke) by the later age of onset, poorer response to treatment, and more marked cognitive and physical impairments. Family and personal history of depression is also less common. Patients may benefit from anti-depressants, but tolerance is often poor.

Other presentations associated with stroke include anxiety, aggression (SSRIs may be of benefit) and fatigue (anti-depressants only of value if co-morbid anxiety and depression).

14.5 Disorders presenting with predominantly physical symptoms

This heading refers to a complex, challenging group of disorders, important for those working in a medical setting where they frequently present. The complexities of the diagnostic classification systems (including differences between DSM-5 and ICD-10) are beyond the remit of this text, other than to note that the terms somatoform disorder and medically unexplained symptoms have been removed from the most recent version of DSM and are likely to be amended in ICD-11. This section will describe some of the **common features** of this group and then focus on conditions specifically described in ICD-10.

Key features of these presentations include:

- **Prominent somatic (physical) symptoms**, e.g. pain, headache, palpitations (feeling their heart beat is abnormal in rate or volume), tremor.

- Symptoms (usually) cause **significant distress** with cognitive, behavioural, and affective responses that perpetuate and worsen their distress.

- Either no underlying **medical pathology** evident or, if present, **does not fully explain** the symptoms and signs.

- Somatic symptoms **cannot be explained by another mental illness**, e.g. depression, anxiety/panic disorder.

Not all disorders presenting with prominent physical symptoms display these characteristics. Patients may also present with physical symptoms, such as limb weakness with little or no distress (conversion disorder). A further (small) subgroup of patients deliberately elaborate or feign mental or physical symptoms (factitious disorder).

Because physical (somatic) symptoms are the main presenting features in these cases, they invariably present in medical settings and may have repeated investigations and procedures, which perpetuate the symptoms, associated beliefs, and distress. As a group, they present huge challenges for the physicians as there is always the concern that an underlying medical condition has been 'missed'. Furthermore, previous labelling of these conditions as 'medically unexplained' often left patients feeling that they were being told there was 'nothing wrong with them'. They are associated, therefore, with significant distress for both treating teams and patients.

A recent shift to focus on symptoms presented and associated beliefs, emotions, and behaviours allows recognition of the patient's distress and provides a guide for psychological intervention.

Predisposing factors may be genetic (e.g. sensitivity to pain) and/or environmental (e.g. family history of attention focused on physical symptoms or physical symptoms as manifestation of distress). There may be a history of childhood adversity. Cultural or social attitudes to physical illness may play a role.

14.5.1 Hypochondriasis (illness anxiety disorder)
Core features (see Clinical vignette Hypochondriasis):

- A persistent belief they have a serious, progressive physical illness that has not been diagnosed.
- Can present with prominent somatic symptoms and a high level of anxiety about their health.
- Repeatedly check themselves or request medical reviews/investigations, none of which provide reassurance.
- Usually a chronic, relapsing/remitting course, presenting in early and middle adulthood.
- Frequent co-morbid disorders (generalized anxiety, depression).

Clinical vignette Hypochondriasis

'Mrs X, a 39-year-old single woman, was convinced she had cancer, probably a rare type that was difficult to diagnose. She had looked up "MEN [multiple endocrine neoplasia] syndrome" on-line and felt her symptoms fitted that diagnosis. She had vague abdominal pain, had lost appetite and weight. She felt tense and on-edge and frequently had facial flushing. She intermittently had diarrhoea. All investigations were normal. In the previous year, she had been concerned she might have a brain tumour, as she had recurrent headaches and felt her vision was blurring. Three years prior to that, her concerns had focused on possible oesophageal cancer, as she felt she had difficulty swallowing, had lost her appetite, and had pains in her chest. In the 5 years prior to her referral, she had been seen by 12 different specialists, had five endoscopies, three CT TAPs, four MRIs, and multiple X-rays and blood tests. All had been normal. Mrs X remained convinced she had an undiagnosed medical illness. She spent considerable time monitoring her symptoms, feeling her pulse regularly, checking her face in the mirror for flushing, and taking her blood pressure using a home monitor. Her symptoms had become completely debilitating. She couldn't think of anything else. She had lost contact with friends and family and knew she was likely to lose her job.' Psychiatrist

---

14.5.1.1 Additional points
- Female = male.
- Prevalence variable.
- Associated with childhood illness.

14.5.1.2 Course and treatment

- Symptoms often persist.
- CBT (see Chapter 16) is of most value in this area, helping the patient to understand and manage their symptoms.
- SSRI may be helpful, particularly if co-morbid depression/anxiety.

14.5.2 Body dysmorphic disorder (BDD)

In ICD-10, this is classified within hypochondriasis (with OCD in DSM). Core features:

- Preoccupation with perceived defects in physical appearance, not obvious to others.
- Significant distress and impairment.
- Often continuously check the perceived defect.
- As with all somatic disorders, these beliefs are strongly held but with some insight.
- If the beliefs are held with no insight, it is considered a delusional disorder (delusional dysmorphophobia).
- CBT may be helpful.
- Antipsychotics, while used (particularly in those with delusional dysmorphophobia) are rarely effective.

14.5.3 Dissociative (conversion) disorders

This group of presentations includes:

- Patients who present with altered **voluntary motor or sensory function** (usually a loss of function, e.g. paralysis or blindness, although they may present with abnormal movements). This was previously termed **hysteria/conversion** disorder.
- Patients who present with disruption of the normal integration of identity and memory (e.g. amnesia), often termed **dissociative disorder** (classified separately in DSM).

These presentations, unconsciously driven, are often acute, dramatic, and represent the patient's idea of how the illness would present. The symptoms and signs usually do not fit with any underlying medical disorder. Frequently, the patient does not display the level of distress one would expect with such a deficit ('*la belle indifférence*'). Historically, the condition was described as occurring in the context of unbearable stress, representing the patient's mechanism for coping or avoiding the underlying stress. Once diagnosed, management (psychological) is focused on support, rehabilitation, and preventing unhelpful reinforcement of the underlying physical symptoms.

14.5.4 Non-epileptic seizures (NES)

NES are generally considered within this group of disorders. Patients present with convulsions that mimic epilepsy. Usually, they do not have the severe physical sequelae, such as tongue-biting, incontinence, and injury due to falls. Management is focused on early identification, limiting of investigations, and support and rehabilitation.

14.5.5 Somatoform autonomic dysfunction (SAD)

ICD-10 includes this disorder, which is characterized by symptoms associated with autonomic arousal, e.g. palpitations, sweating, flushing tremor, etc. These are associated with distress and beliefs about a serious underlying medical disorder. Distinguishing these cases from hypochondriacal disorder (see 14.5.1) can be difficult. A CBT approach is to focus on the predominant symptoms: in hypochondriasis it is the fear of a specific underlying illness, in SAD it is on multiple physical symptoms. DSM, acknowledging the overlaps, has subsumed much of this category into somatic symptom disorders.

14.5.6 Somatization disorder

ICD-10 describes this as recurrent, frequently changing physical symptoms of at least 2 years, with a long and complex medical history. It is associated with disruption of social, interpersonal, and family relations. DSM-5 has subsumed this disorder into somatic symptom disorders.

14.5.7 Persistent somatoform pain disorder

In common with the other disorders presented in this section, this disorder presents with prominent physical symptoms, in this case, pain, which is severe, persistent, distressing, and out of keeping with, or not explained by, underlying medical conditions. As with the other disorders, the patient has very high levels of worry and distress about illness, and the pain may assume a central role in their life and relationships.

This is a particularly complex clinical presentation, as all pain is a subjective sensation, modified by personal sensitivity to pain, affective state, beliefs about the pain, and any co-morbid stressors. Furthermore, the longer that pain persists, the more established it becomes, with some theories suggesting that it can become self-perpetuating. Again, early identification and rehabilitation is key.

14.6 Disorders shaped by medical illness/treatments

14.6.1 Depression in a medical setting

Many features of depression (insomnia, anorexia, weight loss, reduced concentration, energy, and enjoyment—together with a feeling of sadness) are direct consequences of medical illnesses and treatment. Disentangling these physical symptoms from mood can be difficult. It requires careful history-taking, collateral history from family and nursing staff, observation, and sometimes assessment over several visits. As many 'physical' symptoms of depression are unhelpful or misleading, one must rely on 'cognitive' features of depression: lack of enjoyment, lack of hope, lack of interest. Even these can be difficult to judge in a patient who is physically unwell. Questions must be adapted to the patient's state. One may need to ask whether they are able to enjoy visits from their family. Most patients, no matter how unwell, will endorse this. Similarly, while they may not be able to enjoy their usual hobbies, they may still get enjoyment in a more peripheral way—seeing plants in a window-box, following their sport on the television. Finally, even in the most horrific of circumstances, most patients retain hope. A patient who is without hope must be very carefully assessed. If one diagnoses depression, treatment follows the principles discussed in the relevant chapters.

14.6.2 Steroid-induced mood change
See Clinical vignette Steroid-induced mood change.

> **Clinical vignette** Steroid-induced mood change
>
> 'A 54-year-old widow had taken high-dose steroids as part of her lymphoma-protocol. A quiet, reserved lady, with no history of mental illness, she had been absolutely horrified by her experience of steroid-induced mania. She remembered events clearly, describing her disinhibition, impulsive behaviour—actions she deeply regretted. She told of her shame and distress. She was very clear on two points: (1) she would prefer to have cancer again than to ever suffer from mental illness and (2) she asked that all clinicians prescribing steroids be aware of, and counsel patients about, side-effects. She identified [severe] insomnia as the early-warning sign.
>
> 'As a liaison psychiatrist, working with mental illness in a medical setting, I have never forgotten this lady's statements—both her impassioned plea for education about steroids, and her very clear message about the huge burden of mental illness. It is an important message about those who struggle with mental illness.' Liaison Psychiatrist

This disorder is often misleadingly termed **steroid 'psychosis'**—an unhelpful misnomer as the patient is rarely psychotic. Steroids are used in many settings in medicine. Steroid-induced mood changes are common, but often unrecognized. Most commonly, the patient presents with 'hypo'-mania—insomnia, over-talkativeness, and overactivity. Insomnia is the first symptom, an early warning sign. Often the patients will only sleep for 2–3 h at night. Subsequently the patient can become overactive, and chaotic in behaviour, with numerous 'lists' and activities. In keeping with a picture of elevated mood, they can become disinhibited and grandiose, often making phone-calls or decisions they later regret, or impulsively spending. Rarely, it can progress to severe manic symptoms, where the patient can present a danger to themselves. Medical wards, particularly bone-marrow transplant units, are not well placed to manage patients with mania. It is crucial, therefore, to rapidly identify and intervene. As with mania in general psychiatry, patients rarely have clear insight into the disorder, although they may be aware of perpetual restlessness coupled with exhaustion. Encouraging them to take medication and engage in treatment can be difficult and will usually require help from relatives.

It is important when prescribing steroids to inform patients (and their relatives) of the early symptoms (severe insomnia, hyperactivity); and to intervene to prevent deterioration. If steroids must be used (frequently the case), then addition of medication (antipsychotic, e.g. olanzapine) is needed. Benzodiazepines are not effective. The usual considerations of side-effects and drug interactions need to be made (particularly in a medical setting) and, as always, start with a low dose, titrating upwards according to clinical response. Patients usually become aware of the effective dose, often describing a sense of calm and reduction in agitation. When steroids are discontinued, patients may experience a reduction in energy or become low in mood. This is usually self-limiting, but patients are better able to manage this period if informed in advance. Antipsychotics must be reduced in tandem with the reduction in steroids. Occasionally, patients will need anti-depressant treatment. This requires careful consideration if the patient has been manic on steroids. Finally, as always in medicine, in these latter cases, disentangling the low energy, reduced interest and enjoyment due to physical illness/treatment from pervasively low mood can be difficult and will need careful history, examination, and monitoring before adding to the patient's medication list.

14.6.3 Cancer-related fatigue
Many patients with cancer experience profound fatigue. This has many causes:

- Effects of the illness.
- Effects of treatments.
- General de-conditioning due to prolonged periods of being bed-bound.

Patients' recovery is often hampered by advice to 'take it easy' or 'don't do too much' that endorses further rest, worsening de-conditioning. Frequently, after prolonged periods, frustrated by inactivity and sense of powerlessness, patients suddenly try to exercise at 'normal' levels to 'prove' they are fine. These sudden spurts in activity almost inevitably lead to exhaustion, collapse, and further demoralization.

The management of cancer-related fatigue requires careful assessment and joint-working with medical colleagues to define underlying physical contributions, identify any psychiatric co-morbidity (e.g. depression), and the expertise of clinical psychology, physiotherapy, and related disciplines to engage the patient in a gradual return to fitness.

14.7 Disorders presenting with physical symptoms deliberately caused (factitious disorder/Munchausen's)

The concept that a patient would deliberately give themselves physical symptoms to access care is one that is bewildering to many. As the presentation invariably includes deception, it strikes at the heart of the patient–doctor interaction, usually founded on trust, honesty, and mutual respect. Like many complex disorders, there is a spectrum, ranging from exaggeration of existing symptoms (a behaviour that many may endorse) to deliberate causation of symptoms/signs.

Factitious disorder specifically refers to the deliberate production of physical (or psychological) symptoms for **no obvious gain**. The motivation is usually obscure, often linked to the 'gains' of the sick-role. It is distinguished from somatoform disorders (see 14.5), as the physical symptoms are **deliberately**, as opposed to unconsciously, produced. Munchuasen's syndrome, a term often used synonymously with factitious disorder, is a subtype, based on a historical figure, referring to an extreme version, highly dramatic, with presentations to multiple hospitals. Factitious disorder is associated with marked disorder of personality and/or personal relationships, an abusive childhood, and, often, experience of illness within the family or the workplace. Making a diagnosis is very difficult, as it will strike at the heart of the doctor–patient relationship, suggesting to the patient that they are not honest with their teams. Most doctors, unsurprisingly, do not wish to make the diagnosis, both because it is so difficult to be certain, and the consequences can be detrimental to their relationship. However, failing to make the diagnosis will invariably lead to repeated investigations and interventions, escalating risks of harm to the patient, and inappropriate use of scarce resources. Management will require excellent cross-disciplinary team-work and consistent, senior input.

Clinical vignette Factitious disorder

'A 52-year-old single male first presented with a non-healing wound on his left forearm—caused by a farm accident. Despite multiple interventions—antibiotics, repeated excisions, skin-grafts—the wound persisted. There were some unusual features. Typically, the wound improved when the patient was admitted, breaking down once discharged. Microbiology cultivated 'unusual' microbes, pathologists noted 'unusual' particles in skin biopsies. The surgeon was also puzzled. The patient, living in an isolated, impoverished rural setting, seemed relatively unconcerned. He was seen by psychiatry, who noted his impoverished personal circumstances (social, interpersonal, and financial) his relative indifference and lack of psychological-mindedness, but did not identify any major mental illness. A large meeting of multiple teams was held (plastics, infectious diseases, microbiology, dermatology, and psychiatry). The possibility of factitious disorder was raised, but other than atypical features, there was no evidence to support this. A discussion with the patient about possible causes,

continued >

including "inadvertent" interference with the wound, led to vigorous denial. A decision was made to include psychological medicine in management, focusing on rehabilitation and social engagement.

'Weeks later, following further surgery, the patient suddenly stopped passing urine into his catheter bag post-operatively and developed severe abdominal pain. Emergency urology assessment, renal ultrasound, and bloods did not reveal any abnormality. The catheter bag remained empty. Some hours later, a nurse found a large bowl of urine under the patient's bed. The patient was unable to explain how it was there. The bowl was removed, constant observation by nursing staff was put in place, and the patient began to pass urine into the catheter bag.

'Further meetings, between teams and with the patient, suggested that the patient could not always be honest with staff—something that the patient broadly accepted, though not in relation to his wound. A complex management strategy was implemented with the aim of limiting further surgical interventions and promoting psychological well-being. The family remained resolutely opposed to the concept that the patient might be in any way responsible for his presentation.' Psychiatrist

The Clinical vignette Factitious disorder exhibits many of the key features of factitious disorder: initial, prolonged search for medical/surgical causes; reluctance to consider factitious disorder; resolute denial by the patient; anger and disbelief from the family. It also illustrates a way of management—sharing of expertise with colleagues in making a diagnosis, focus on identifying a single piece of evidence that supported the diagnosis, and a management plan that involved multiple team members providing support and focus on recovery.

14.8 Malingering

It is with some reluctance that this heading is included in a handbook on mental illness. In malingering, people deliberately, consciously, feign illness but the aim is very clearly focused on material gain—financial or legal. Making this deduction, in cases often embroiled in complex legal cases, requires skills at the level of actual detectives and generally should be left within that sphere. These cases, by definition, do not have a mental illness.

14.9 Interventions in liaison

Many of the presentations in liaison are complex, requiring multi-disciplinary assessment and implementation of combined psychological, biological, and social interventions. As many of the patients are physically ill, on multiple medications, medication must be scrupulously selected, if needed. Psychological interventions exist on a spectrum of complexity—the intervention should be matched to the need. A model to develop and deliver this service is presented in Chapter 16 (Figure 16.1).

14.10 Summary

Psychological medicine/liaison psychiatry represents the interface between physical and mental health. Presentations will include delirium, dementia, self-harm, and substance abuse—all discussed in relevant chapters. This chapter has focused on conditions where patients either present with physical symptoms not explained by an underlying medical condition, or with medical conditions, particularly neurological conditions, such as Parkinson's disease or epilepsy, associated with significant mental health burden. The service's broadest remit—supporting colleagues in medicine and surgery caring for patients with complex mental and physical health-needs—permeates all aspects of any well-embedded service.

CHAPTER 15

Forensic perspectives in general psychiatry

CHAPTER FOCUS
What you should know about forensic psychiatry
• The principles of consent to treatment.
• The principles of treatment without consent.
• Concepts of 'risk' and professional judgement.

15.1 Introduction

Legal aspects of mental health are complex, with far-reaching implications for patients and clinicians. While some legal aspects of medical care require the intervention of specialists in psychiatry and the law (forensic psychiatrists), every doctor will encounter, and needs to manage, legal aspects of medical and psychiatric care in their daily work. While every jurisdiction has specific laws, common concepts exist across all jurisdictions. This introductory guide for medical students, accordingly, will focus on subjects that any doctor is likely to encounter, namely:

- Capacity (and legislation).
- Consent.
- Risk.

Confidentiality is reviewed in Chapters 1 and 19.

15.2 Capacity

15.2.1 Capacity to consent

The issue of whether a patient has capacity to consent to an intervention regularly arises for all doctors, not just psychiatrists. It is an important issue, as proceeding to any intervention without the patient's consent can be interpreted as an assault.

To fully consent to an intervention, the patient must be able to:

- **Understand** the information fully:
  - ○ Why the treatment is being carried out.
  - ○ The risks/benefits of having OR not having the procedure.

- **Retain** this information.
- **Evaluate** the information to make an informed decision ('weigh up' the information).
- **Communicate** their decision.
- **Not** be under **duress** with respect to the decision.

Note:

- **Everyone** has capacity until proven otherwise.
- The presence of a **mental illness** does **NOT** necessarily mean the patient lacks capacity.
- Capacity assessments are **specific** to each task. One cannot say 'the patient has capacity'. Instead one says, for example, 'the patient has capacity to consent to bowel resection'.
- Every patient, with capacity, has the **right to refuse** treatment. People can, and do, regularly make unwise decisions in everyday life, as well as in health.

Engaging the patient to assess consent, particularly in the context of emergency departments, can be difficult. It requires calm, quietness, and time—ingredients often in short supply in these settings. However, stopping to engage with the patient, to establish rapport, and to clarify consent are crucial to good patient care (see Clinical vignette Consent).

Clinical vignette Consent

'Soon after starting as a psychiatry trainee, I was called to the Emergency Department at 3 a.m. A 21-year-old single female needed an intravenous infusion of acetylcysteine for a paracetamol overdose, without which she risked fulminant liver failure. The patient was agitated, screaming, and shouting, refusing all treatment, threatening to leave. The ED team wanted to proceed to give her the infusion against her will, judging her to lack capacity, and deeming the intervention urgent as the "cut-off" time to administer the drug was close.

'On my way to the ED, I wondered about judging someone, who did not have any obvious mental illness, as lacking capacity. I thought about the practicalities of giving an IV infusion over several hours to a physically able, agitated person who did not want it. I worried about the consequences of her refusing treatment, or leaving the department.

'When I arrived at the ED, there was chaos. The young woman was in a corner, shouting, crying, screaming abuse, refusing to allow anyone near her.

'It took almost an hour—of persuading her to move into a quiet space, asking her to sit down, listening to her story without interruption. But, ultimately, she

continued >

---

agreed to treatment. And while it took a long time, I learned a valuable lesson that evening. It was time worth spending. The alternatives—making decisions about lack of capacity, proceeding to treatment, and an IV-infusion without consent—were impossible.' Consultant Psychiatrist

15.2.2 Treatment without consent

No doctor should ever wish to proceed without consent of their patient. This is both a practical and an ethical statement. It is effectively impossible to proceed with most interventions without the consent of your patient. If you do proceed, subsequent lack of consent/co-operation is likely to render the intervention unsuccessful. More importantly, ethically, it transgresses every tenet of the doctor–patient relationship to proceed without consent. Finally, proceeding without consent can constitute assault.

It is, however, inevitable that, despite following all the guidelines, you will be faced with a situation where a patient refuses an intervention you deem essential. Doctors generally find these situations very unsettling, as most doctors are accustomed to their patients' agreeing to interventions they believe they are suggesting in good faith.

There are several important considerations. First, carefully:

- Re-assess the process, engage with the patient.
- If this is unsuccessful, assess the patient's capacity for the specific decision using the procedure discussed. Everyone has the right to make unwise decisions if they have capacity to do so.
- Consider the implications of the decision being made. A decision with minor consequences (e.g. a decision to paint their house red) is less likely to need activation of legal aid (other than noting it lest it be an indicator of future deterioration), compared to a decision to refuse life-saving treatment.
- Assess for mental illness. A person may have a mental illness and still retain capacity. However, if the mental illness directly influences the decision being made, then treatment of the mental illness (under **mental health legislation**) may be needed with subsequent review of consent for the physical procedure.

Practical tips Treatment without consent

- It is much, much better to proceed with the patient's consent—always endeavour to achieve this.
- Take time gathering information before seeing the patient.
- Take time sitting with the patient, hearing their story, and clarifying any misconceptions.

continued >

- Consider options other than proceeding with treatment.
- If treatment is necessary, and patient lacks capacity, ensure the patient receives the appropriate treatment as compassionately as possible.

Inevitably, despite all these interventions, there will be situations where you must proceed to treatment without consent. Where possible, you should always consult with colleagues (and legal advisors) in these situations. (See Practical tips Treatment without consent.)

Treatment without consent is likely to fall under one of four categories.

15.2.2.1 Emergency interventions: 'common law'

'Common law' refers to principles of law within a jurisdiction, derived from custom and practice, shaped by court judgements (and, therefore, subject to change). It supports a doctor's 'duty of care' and includes concepts of:

- Reasonableness (what any reasonable doctor would do in this situation).
- Necessity (to prevent death/serious harm).
- Acting in accordance with a recognized body of opinion.
- A logical, defensible process.

Examples of interventions under common law:

- An **emergency life-threatening situation,** where the patient is unable to consent (e.g. unconscious). In these difficult circumstances the clinician may need to proceed without consent as 'necessity' under 'common law' to fulfil a duty of care. The doctor should still strive to:
  - O Get a second opinion.
  - O Consult with the family (although a family member can NOT consent on behalf of a patient).
- Treatment for **acute behavioural disturbance** due to suspected mental or physical illness (again treated as '**necessity**' under 'common law' to fulfil a duty of care, pending review under the **Mental Health Act**).

15.2.2.2 Treatment of mental illness under the relevant jurisdiction's mental health laws

Many jurisdictions have developed specific legislation for patients who need treatment for, but lack capacity due to, mental illness. These mental health laws (Acts) are specific for each jurisdiction but share commonalities:

- Allow detention of patients in approved mental health centres for assessment and/or treatment of mental disorder.
- For specified periods only.

- Must be reviewed by independent panel of experts.
- Compulsory treatment of mental disorder under specific restrictions (medication only, must be reviewed by independent psychiatrist following a certain period, other treatments, e.g. ECT, psycho-surgery, require additional independent assessment).
- Limited to treatment of mental disorder only (physical treatments unrelated to the mental disorder are excluded).

The admission (and treatment) of a patient against their will (**involuntary detention**), and the associated deprivation of liberty, is a serious breach of that person's civil liberties. It is a very difficult decision for any clinician and is only taken after careful consideration and in the context of the relevant Mental Health Act (MHA). Equally, however, failure to care for a person with severe mental illness who is lacking insight and whose judgement is impaired and is, therefore, unable to seek treatment, is a gross violation of that person's right to care and can have serious adverse outcomes not only for themselves but also others.

Psychiatrists must be familiar with specific mental health laws in their own jurisdictions. As newly qualified doctors, you will need to be aware of the common principles including:

- Acting in the best interest of the person.
- Regard to safety of the person and others.
- Safe-guarding of the person's rights, including right to dignity, privacy, and autonomy (with right to appeal the process).

The Acts also generally provide:

- Definitions of mental disorder.
- Specific criteria for compulsory detention.

As a 'general' doctor, you may be asked to provide a **medical assessment** in response to an application for involuntary admission (e.g. by spouse, relative, authorized officer, member of police) to state whether you believe the person may have a mental disorder, supporting a recommendation for admission for assessment or treatment. Specific guidance in each situation is available on the websites of the relevant jurisdiction (e.g. irishstatutebook.ie). Always **consult your colleagues if unclear**.

15.2.2.3 Treatment under specific capacity legislation

Several jurisdictions have recently introduced specific laws relating to capacity. If you are involved in a capacity case, you will need to be familiar with laws within the jurisdiction in which you are operating. Examples of Capacity Acts, outlined for general information below, share common themes, largely reflecting the points raised when discussing capacity.

The **Mental Capacity Act (2005) (England and Wales)** seeks to support vulnerable individuals, outlining how to assess for capacity and how to make decisions in their best interest. This Act also allows for **advance decisions** (made by someone with capacity) to refuse treatment in the future (except those deemed to be needed for comfort, e.g. offering food/drink by mouth) and to appoint an attorney to act on their behalf if they lose capacity in the future (**lasting power of attorney**). Safeguards include a court of protection, public guardians, and independent mental capacity advocates.

Adults with Incapacity Act (2000) (Scotland) governs decisions made in the best interest of persons with impaired capacity considering the person's wishes, benefits, existing capacity, and relevant others. It includes power of attorney for welfare, finances, and medical treatments

The **Mental Capacity Act (2016) (Northern Ireland)** combines both mental capacity and mental health law under one Act and has been partially implemented since December 2019. It upholds the principles of capacity outlined above (decision-specific, capacity presumed, allowing unwise decisions).

The **Assisted Decision-Making (Capacity) Act (2015) (Ireland)** (partially commenced) outlines a graded approach to capacity/decision-making ranging from assisted, co-decision, to decision-making representative. It allows for enduring powers of attorney to include welfare and introduces advanced healthcare directives, made by the individual while they had capacity, signed by two witnesses and a designated healthcare representative (if appointed), and applicable if the person lacks capacity at the time of the intervention regarding that specific intervention.

15.2.2.4 Specific judgements applied from court

Occasionally, the clinician will need to seek specific direction from the Courts for an individual case. These cases may then be subsumed into 'common law'.

15.2.3 Testamentary capacity

This is a subtype of capacity, referring to capacity to make a will. The same factors for capacity to consent apply, with the **additional need** for the person to know:

- The extent and value of their property.
- Their natural beneficiaries.
- What they are leaving and to whom.

15.3 **Risk assessment**

Any doctor may be asked to give an opinion about 'risk'—of harm to self or others (typically in the Emergency Department). Those of you who become psychiatrists will be asked for opinions in more complex areas.

As discussed in Chapter 1, the terms 'risk' and 'risk assessment' have crept into use in medical assessments, frequently included as 'boxes' to be 'ticked'. Yet 'risk', by definition, refers to the future—possibility/chance/likelihood of an adverse event. Doctors cannot predict the future. What we can do, however, is use assessment to identify factors that **increase the likelihood** of an adverse event, and consider **ways to mitigate** these factors.

Several 'risk' factors may be **unamenable to intervention** (e.g. previous history of violence, young age, male gender). Others, such as co-morbid substance abuse, poor social support, and fractured relationships, while they may be amenable to intervention, provide huge challenges to change. For others, however, (e.g. acute psychosis with auditory hallucinations or delusions promoting self-harm or harm to others) psychiatrists can play a valuable role in treating these factors that increase risk and may be **amenable to intervention**.

The importance (and urgency) of a risk assessment depends on the **likelihood** and **seriousness** of the potential outcome—both often hard to judge. Violence-to-self (suicide) or others is, perhaps, the most extreme example of a serious outcome. Many 'risk assessments' are focused on these areas. As these assessments focus on predicting the future, they run the risk of **false-positive** results (wrongly suggesting the person will engage in violent acts) leading to **unnecessarily treating or detaining** the person. Alternatively, they can lead to **false-negative** results (wrongly suggesting the person won't engage in violent acts) with the **risk of serious violence** to self or others as an outcome. Most clinicians are likely to err on the side of caution with higher false-positive results (and low false-negative results).

However, because in many cases (particularly, for example, emergency presentations with deliberate self-harm) the **absolute risk** of a serious adverse event is very low, and the **number of factors predicting risk** are often both **very high** (young, males, history of co-morbid substance abuse, adverse early childhood, poor social supports) and **very difficult to treat** (as already discussed), many clinicians assessing emergency psychiatry presentations are faced with very challenging situations. Furthermore, the 'interventions' available are often very limited, with many factors not amenable to change, certainly in the short-term. The concept that 'admission' will inevitably reduce the risk and will not result in any harm is not true. It is also not available for the numbers presenting to Emergency Departments. Recurrent admissions can impair patients' ability to learn to manage crises and develop their own strategies. Admissions of people with challenging behaviours, such as violence and drug-use, occurring outside the context of mental illness, introduces chaos and disruption for the other in-patients with serious mental illness (see also Chapters 2, 6, and 18 and Figure 15.1).

15.3.1 Structured professional judgement (SPJ)
Forensic psychiatry acknowledges the difficulties with respect to 'risk' and uses a 'structured professional judgement' tool in assessment. This tool uses both

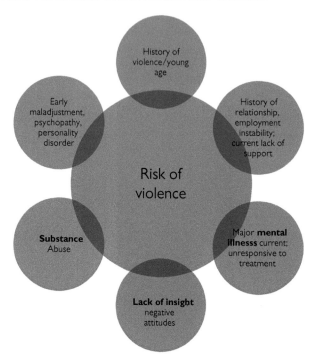

Figure 15.1 Some of the complex, inter-linked factors within the patient—historical, clinical, current—that amplify risk of violence.

clinical judgement and research-based evidence. It **acknowledges several important factors:**

- Risk is dynamic and varies over time.
- Factors that contribute to risk include both static and dynamic factors.
- The focus is, therefore, on planning management rather than 'predicting dangerousness'.
- The seriousness of the situation (so-called 'high risk scenarios') will influence management.

15.3.1.1 HCR-20

The **HCR-20** is a well-established SPJ tool. It looks at **historical items** associated with adverse outcomes:

- Previous violence.
- Young age at first violent incident.

- Relationship instability.
- Employment difficulties.
- Substance misuse.
- Major mental illness.
- Psychopathy.
- Early maladjustment.
- Personality disorder.
- Previous supervision failure.

Also **clinical** items:

- Lack of insight.
- Negative attitudes.
- Active symptoms of mental illness.
- Impulsivity.
- Unresponsive to treatment.

It also looks at factors in the **management plan** that will increase risk:

- Lacks feasibility.
- Ongoing exposure to destabilizers.
- Lack of personal support.
- Non-compliance with remediation attempts.
- Stress.

The SPJ tool also helps in **charting progress** in treatment and recovery in a forensic context and triage for levels of care.

Shorter term assessment tools, such as the **DASA** (dynamic appraisal of situational aggression), aim to rate **risk of aggression** on a day-to-day basis, generally in in-patient units. These chart behaviours such as irritability, impulsivity, unwillingness to follow directions, sensitivity to perceived provocation, easily angered when requests are denied, negative attitudes, and verbal threats. As with any tool of assessment, it must be used **within the context of clinical judgement** and is not prescriptive.

The context in which these tools are used is very important. Many of the forensic assessments will be **elective**, done **over long periods of time**, the subjects usually **in-patients in safe, controlled environments.** Many of the (emergency) assessments in psychiatry will be **emergencies**, done **over brief periods of time,** with the subjects usually in **Emergency Departments**, in **busy, chaotic environments**, often with little or no ability to gain collateral or detailed previous history. The clinical VIGNETTE 'Risk' assessment in ED—two different outcomes illustrates some of these issues.

> **Clinical vignettes** 'Risk' assessment in ED—two different outcomes
>
> 'A 24-year-old single man was brought to the ED by ambulance. He had been wandering the streets, shouting, and agitated, and was noted to be bleeding from both forearms. On assessment in the ED, he had multiple lacerations on both forearms, some of which required suturing. He was agitated throughout the assessment, shouting at "voices" he could hear that were telling him to kill himself, that he was a bad person. He was very afraid, convinced "bad people" were out to get him. He had no known prior history of mental illness, denied drug abuse, and his urine toxicology screen was clear. He was physically well. No collateral history was available, as he refused to give contact details. He was judged to be acutely psychotic, posing a risk to himself in responding to his psychotic symptoms, and was admitted for urgent psychiatric assessment under the Mental Health Act.
>
> 'Later that evening, a 21-year-old single woman was brought to the ED by ambulance. She also was wandering the streets, shouting, and agitated, shouting that she was going to cut herself. She was noted to have several cuts to her forearms. On assessment, she had multiple superficial lacerations on both forearms, with multiple, healed scars. She was tearful and distressed, saying she could not cope. She was well-known in the ED, regularly presenting out-of-hours in a distressed state. She had a long history of self-cutting and attended the local community mental health team for regular support with a diagnosis of emotionally unstable personality disorder. She had had 18 admissions over the previous 3 years, in the context of self-harm. She had started a psychological treatment (dialectical behaviour therapy) with the aim of supporting her in managing her crises outside of hospital, learning to live independently, while managing her distress. After careful reading of her case history and treatment plans, the psychiatrist-on-call spent a considerable time with the patient discussing her management plans and alternative safety plans to admission. She was ultimately discharged to the care of a relative, with a plan for urgent review by her team the next morning.' Consultant emergency medicine

'Risk' or adverse future events, can never be eliminated. Nevertheless, **with the aim of intervening when possible, the concept of identifying items that may increase risk, and factors that are likely to hamper safe management, forms a good basis for clinical assessment.**

15.4 Summary

Some legal aspects of psychiatry are complex, requiring the input of specialist forensic psychiatrists. However, there are several areas with which all doctors (and medical students) should be familiar, as they include situations with which they will be faced, regularly, during their practice. These include judgements about capacity, including consent, confidentiality 'risk', and broad aspects of mental health legislation that allow for the care of patients with mental illness.

CHAPTER 16

Psychological treatments

CHAPTER FOCUS

What you should know about psychological treatments
- The role of the MDT.
- Psycho-education.
- Psycho-therapy—common and specific elements.
- How BT and CBT work.
- Examples of cognitive distortions and how they affect mental state.

16.1 Introduction: general principles

A bio-psycho-social approach helps to define management—usually psycho-social interventions delivered by a multi-disciplinary team (MDT) and medication, when appropriate.

This chapter focuses on psychological interventions and the MDT. Chapter 17 focuses on physical interventions. They are not exhaustive but, in keeping with the aims of this handbook, focus on important concepts you are likely to encounter (and use) while working in medicine outside psychiatry.

16.2 The multi-disciplinary team (MDT)

Mental healthcare should be delivered by a multi-disciplinary team—psychiatrists, mental health nurses, social workers, occupational therapists, (clinical) psychologists, and others, e.g. pharmacists. The team works with patients and their supports (family, friends, and community).
A good MDT brings:

- Differing professional perspectives.
- Collaborative assessments.
- Combined expertise.
- Peer-support.

Challenges for MDTs include:

- Lack of resources.
- Poor team-working.
- Lack of understanding of members' roles.

Like any area, to function well, an MDT requires continuous care and review. A well-functioning MDT helps to optimize patient care—directly, by providing a range of interventions and expertise, and, indirectly, by supporting team members (see Clinical vignette MDT).

Clinical vignette MDT

'While this placement has had many challenging moments, it has most made me appreciate the importance of positive team dynamics. When I think about the MDT in this service, the following come to mind:

- Leadership: consultants take interest not only in clinical matters, but also are vigilant about the well-being of staff (e.g. mindful of workload, supporting staff dealing with physical health issues) and are always available.
- Respect: no matter what the grade/position of the team member, a mutual respect is always shown, opinions are sought from everyone.
- Closeness, support, and collaboration: it actually feels like a team with different specialities working together for a common goal. Everyone is doing their part but the overall picture is not lost because of good communication. People proactively enquire whether others need help.
- Expertise and experience: most team members are long-term, they have built an amazing skillset, and continue enriching it by learning from each other. It also means there is continuity for patients, even in a liaison setting.
- Humour: it makes the challenges of the work (which can be difficult at times) less daunting.' Liaison Psychiatry Trainee

---

16.2.1 MDT members

16.2.1.1 Occupational therapy (OT)

- Provides functional assessments on:
  o Self-care, productivity, and leisure activities.
- Supports performance.
- Promotes recovery (supports balance and routine in patients' lives).

16.2.1.2 Mental health nursing

- Frequently the 'linchpin' of the mental health team.
- Provide continuity of care and expertise at a senior clinical level.
- Contribute to service management and development.

16.2.1.3 Mental health social worker

- Works on behalf of patients with statutory and voluntary organizations.
- Provides support.

- Promotes social inclusion and justice.
- Contributes to the team and service development.

16.2.1.4 (Clinical) psychology

- Key members of MDT.
- Provide assessments and complex psychological interventions.
- Contribute to team perspectives and development.
- Provide support and supervision for other team members delivering psycho-therapy at a less complex level.

16.2.1.5 Psychiatrists

Consultant and junior doctors-in-training provide:

- Broad assessments and interventions (psychological and physical).
- Maintain and develop the service.
- Support the MDT.

16.3 What is psycho-therapy?

At its simplest, psycho-therapy is any intervention that aims to help a person's psychological distress using psychological techniques. Typically, this involves 'words' (talking, listening, and reflecting), but set within a specific framework.

Psychotherapies may be classified according to:

- The **number** of patients taking part (individual, couple, small or large group).
- The **principles** on which they are based (behavioural, cognitive behavioural, psycho-dynamic, etc.).

16.4 Why understand psycho-therapies?

Even though many of you will never use specific psycho-therapy, an understanding of the principles optimizes your care of patients by helping you to:

- More meaningfully engage with colleagues to whom you refer for psychological treatments.
- Refer for appropriate intervention, allowing matching of patients' needs to appropriate interventions, and best use of resources.
- Extract some elements for use yourself in your management of patients and families.
- Reflect on your own practice experiences.

16.5 Model for psycho-therapy delivery

There are several 'levels' (and types) of psycho-therapy. The complexity of the intervention (and expertise needed) should match the level of need. Interventions that are too complex are not only wasteful of a scarce resource, but can be harmful. The model developed by O'Dwyer and Collier (St. James's Hospital, Dublin) for cancer care, incorporated into the National Cancer Control Programme (Ireland), provides a template for delivering psycho-therapy in any medical setting (Figure 16.1). It reflects the spectrum of presentations, matched to interventions, ranging from support to complex psycho-therapies. Furthermore, experts at the bottom of the pyramid provide support, education, and guidance for those at higher levels.

16.6 Psycho-education

Psycho-education refers to the giving of information about mental illness to:

- Patients.
- Families.
- Society.

Distress	Patient Numbers and Levels	Intervention	Provider
Transient, Mild	Level 1	Education (family, patient)	Medical Teams
Persistent Mild	Level 2	Specific psycho education	Medical Team (CNS)
Moderate	Level 3	Simple Psychological Rx	CNS, SW (Mental Health)
Severe (Clinical Disorders)	Level 4	Complex Psychological Rx, and/or medication	Clinical Psychology and Psychiatry
Organic States/Psychosis Suicidality	Level 5	Medication	Psychiatry

Figure 16.1 St. James's model for delivery of psychological care in medical settings.
Reproduced courtesy of St James's Hospital.

It aims to:

- **Empower** patients by giving them an understanding of what is happening.
- **Educate** patients about their illness and treatments, to promote recovery.
- **Educate** the public to combat stigma.

16.6.1 Examples of psycho-education
For patients:

- Simple interventions in mild distress, e.g. explanation of the 'fight-or-flight' concept in anxiety (see Chapter 8).
- Educating patients about symptoms in complex diagnoses, such as schizophrenia.
- Explaining treatments.
- Discussing impact of illness.

For public:

- Aims to inform the public about the impact of mental illness and to reduce stigma (people with mental illness are still **judged** negatively due to their illness). **Shame** and **isolation** are still experienced by many, reducing the likelihood they will seek help, increasing isolation, and despair.
- Students and doctors play a major role in combating stigma and mental health. **Asking about, and acknowledging, mental health** as part of the medical assessment is an important step.
- For those doctors who themselves become mentally ill, the stigma that persists critically reduces the ability of this potentially vulnerable group to seek help (see Chapter 18).

16.7 Common elements of all psychological treatments

The goal of all psychological treatments is to support and to educate patients about their psychological responses, empowering them to, ultimately, effect change themselves.

Common to all psychotherapies, therefore, is the provision of:

- A **safe environment** where they can tell their story.
- A **rationale** for how they are feeling and how they might change this.
- Aids to **promote self-esteem** and acknowledge distress.
- A **respectful, safe,** therapeutic **relationship.**
- A therapist who **listens** and **reflects** on what is being said.

The patient–therapist relationship, a key factor in any patient–doctor interaction, is particularly important in psychological treatments. Given the emotional and highly personal interactions between patient and therapist, the patient may develop 'transference', attributing to the therapist attitudes and feelings that actually reflect their own close relationships. Similarly, the therapist, even while focused on remaining impartial, while being empathic, may project attitudes and behaviours that reflect their own personal relationships, a process called **counter-transference**. The degree to which these reactions are used in therapy varies. They are a central part, for example, of psycho-analytic psycho-therapy. Nonetheless, elements of these reactions are likely to be present in every interaction and therapists should be aware of them, both for the best care of the patient, and for themselves. These seemingly 'simple' interactions require a complex mix of knowledge, skills, and attitudes and are discussed throughout the book.

These features are largely evident in individual therapies. **Group therapies** provide other, common features, which include:

- A sense of **belonging.**
- The ability to learn from their interactions within the group (**interpersonal learning**).
- Learning new behaviours from others (**modelling**).
- Realization that other people have similar problems (**universality**).

Much discussion still exists in the literature on the relative effectiveness of each of the psycho-therapies and which component of therapy is essential. The concept that all therapies share their effectiveness through common factors is known as the 'Dodo bird verdict' (from the Dodo bird in the novel Alice in Wonderland who declared that everyone was a winner in a race, irrespective of results). Researchers (and clinicians) delivering therapies such as behavioural therapy (BT) and cognitive behavioural therapy (CBT) strongly contest this and argue that these treatments produce better clinical effects than others and cite therapy-specific interventions (e.g. exposure therapy in BT). Nonetheless, the therapist–patient relationship (the therapeutic alliance) is crucial, irrespective of the methods used, as without patient engagement, no therapy can proceed effectively.

16.8 Specific elements of psycho-therapies

16.8.1 Psycho-dynamic psycho-therapy and defence mechanisms

While psycho-dynamic psycho-therapy is highly specialized (and a detailed discussion is outside the scope of this book), many processes first described by (Sigmund) Freud are still considered in psycho-therapeutic interactions. Freud believed that all processes originate in the unconscious and that behaviours reflect unconscious struggles between the unconscious and the conscious. He called these unconscious processes **defence mechanisms** and suggested that they are important, not only in the understanding of neurosis, but also in our everyday behaviours. Examples of these defence mechanisms, used in many medical settings, are:

- **Denial:** a person behaves as though they are unaware of what they have been told (e.g. that they are entering a terminal stage of their illness).
- **Sublimation:** unacceptable impulses, e.g. aggressive urges, are turned into vigorous activities, such as chopping firewood, or a need to be always in control, into a role as entrepreneur.
- **Projection:** people attribute to other people emotions they are experiencing themselves, e.g. if they feel angry with a colleague, instead they view the colleague as being angry with them.
- **Regression:** use of behaviour found in an earlier stage of development, e.g. development of child-like dependency in illness.
- **Rationalization:** use of more acceptable explanations for behaviours rather than facing true, more unpalatable ones. For example, someone who spends the last of their limited budget on a camper-van may say this was 'essential' during the Covid-pandemic.

16.8.2 Conditioning and early behavioural interventions
The early building blocks for BT (behavioural therapy) had been established in the 1800s by physiologists. Building on earlier work, Pavlov, a Russian physiologist, sought to provide a scientific explanation for the relationship between physical and psychological acts. Pavlov's work on conditioned reflexes (**'classical' or 'Pavlovian' conditioning**) formed the basis for many of the concepts of **behavioural therapy** (see Table 16.1).

Other behavioural interventions focused on responses that were not initially in the repertoire of the organism under study. This work formed the basis of **operant conditioning**, developed further by an American psychologist B. F. Skinner who described concepts such as *positive reinforcement* (increase in behaviour with reward) and *negative reinforcement* (increase in behaviour with avoidance of an unpleasant event). He also described *aversive conditioning* (an intervention that caused a reduction in behaviour) and *frustrative non-reward* (behaviour not followed by anticipated reward). These ideas were developed further in the USA. A **token economy** system was introduced by Allyon and Azrin, providing patients with tokens to motivate them to do specific tasks that could then be exchanged for real items the person wanted.

16.8.3 Introduction of behavioural therapy
In 1920, Watson and Rayner, using the ideas of Pavlov, artificially conditioned fear of an animal in an 11-month-old child, Albert. They suggested that learning could account for the development of abnormal fear (anxiety) in humans and that

Table 16.1 Classical (Pavlovian) conditioning concepts

Dog	+	Unconditioned stimulus (Food)	+	–		=	Unconditioned response (Salivation)
Dog	+	------------	+	Neutral stimulus (Bell)		=	No response
Repeated pairing of unconditioned and neutral stimulus							
Dog	+	Food	+ (repeatedly)	Bell		=	Salivation
		Leads to:		Conditioned stimulus			Conditioned response
Dog	+	----------	+	Bell		=	Salivation
Dog	+	----------	+	A sound like a bell		=	Salivation (stimulus generalization)
Dog	+	----------	+	A sound unlike a bell		=	No response (Stimulus differentiation)
Dog	+	----------	+ (repeatedly)	Bell (no food)		=	No response (stimulus extinction)

conditioning provided a useful model to study this. These ideas were further developed by Joseph **Wolpe** who worked on the production and elimination of fear in animals (cats). He noted that feeding inhibits anxiety (**reciprocal inhibition**). He suggested that a response antagonistic to anxiety, made repeatedly in the presence of anxiety-provoking stimuli, would weaken the bond between the anxiety response and the stimulus. He also developed the concept of presentation of the feared situation in a hierarchical fashion (**graded exposure**). He extended this principle of reciprocal inhibition from animals to treat neurosis in humans, incorporating an 'inhibitory' technique (progressive muscular relaxation). The most frequently used technique was a combination of hierarchical presentation of the fear-inducing situation, presented in the imagination, together with progressive muscular relaxation (**systematic desensitization**).

Wolpe's contribution was a landmark one from several perspectives. As with Pavlov, it was based on scientific principles derived from the objective observation of behavioural experiments. It combined learning concepts with a neurophysiological understanding of behaviour. The treatment was specific, relatively brief, and measurable. It proposed several hypotheses, each of which was testable and included data on effectiveness. These features were a radical departure from the ideas and techniques of psycho-analysis, which had been the main intervention until that time. In the UK, at the Institute of Psychiatry in London, the development of behavioural therapy gathered momentum with the arrival of Rachman, a student of Wolpe's from South Africa, who worked with Marks, Gelder, and de Silva. Based on the principles described above, they investigated **behavioural therapy** techniques, such as **desensitization, flooding, modelling,** and **aversion therapy**. These techniques were then applied to a variety of disorders, particularly specific phobias, agoraphobia, and obsessive–compulsive disorder. Success rates varied and the identification of the most effective component of the therapy was slow. **Exposure** (to the feared object) proved to be the most important, with graded exposure *in vivo* (and without relaxation) proposed by Marks as the key concepts. The manner of exposure and the **grading of the hierarchy** are key in the therapy (see Marks, Isaac for further detail).

16.8.4 Cognitive behavioural therapy (CBT)

While behavioural therapy led to significant successes in the treatment of disorders such as phobias and OCD, it did not help all conditions. The limitations of an approach that only considered directly observable behaviour were acknowledged. The importance of thought process in behaviour emerged as important concepts.

CBT was first described by Aaron Beck for the treatment of depression. He revolutionized the concepts behind depression suggesting that, **rather than depression causing negative (pessimistic, unhelpful) thoughts, negative thoughts themselves could lead to a depressed mood**. These negative thoughts (thinking errors; see Table 16.2) are usually generated by faulty thinking patterns (cognitive distortions or errors) that reinforce and perpetuate the negative thoughts.

While many people experience these thoughts occasionally, in depression they are persistent and pervasive. Beck suggested that identifying and challenging these unhelpful thoughts (termed negative automatic thoughts, NATS) could both prevent and treat depression (and, later, other disorders). Christine Padesky developed these concepts further, scrutinizing the interaction between thoughts, emotions, behaviours, and physical (body) sensations—often termed the 'hot-cross bun' model (Figure 16.2).

At a more profound level, assessment of early experiences to understand from where these negative styles have arisen (**schema-focused therapy**) can be used, e.g. harsh parenting styles leading to core beliefs of worthlessness.

Getting patients to visualize their problems using this model, showing them how to stop the 'vicious circle' is the first step to engagement and empowering patients to bring about change.

Other facets echo many of the original components of BT:

- Collaboration.
- Problem/solution focus.

Table 16.2 Examples of thinking errors (cognitive distortions)

Thinking error	Explanation	Underlying thoughts (NATS—negative automatic thoughts)
Catastrophization	Predicting the worst will happen, with disastrous consequences	I will fail this exam, and it will ruin my career
Black and white thinking	'All-or-nothing' thinking,	Things are either 'wonderful' or 'disastrous'
Arbitrary inference (jumping to conclusions)	Drawing (negative) conclusions with very little, if any, evidence.	William's girlfriend doesn't reply immediately to his text. He decides she is bored with him and is planning on breaking up.
Selective abstraction/ mental filter	Focus on specific (generally negative) aspects	Feedback on a presentation mainly positive but focuses on one negative comment, decides was a disaster
Overgeneralization	Draws faulty conclusions from a single incident	John is unsuccessful at a job interview. Decides that he will never get a job.
Personalization	Relates events to themselves when there is little evidence for doing so	A work colleague fails to respond to a greeting. Believes was a deliberate snub, triggers other thoughts such as 'no one likes me'

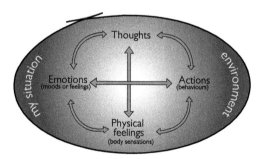

Figure 16.2 **The 'hot-cross bun' model in CBT.**

Reproduced with permission from S Collier and O Dwyer AM, *Cancer-Related Fatigue Manual*, St James's Hospital. Source: Data from Greenberger D and Padesky C (1995) *Mind Over Mood: Changing How You Feel by Changing the Way You Think*, Guildford: Guilford Press.

- Use of behavioural experiments.
- Identification of goals.
- Brief interventions.
- The importance of measurement.

16.8.5 Newer psychological interventions

As with psycho-dynamic psycho-therapy and BT, while CBT enjoyed huge popularity and success, ultimately it was recognized that it was not a panacea, and newer psycho-therapies were developed, e.g. 'third-wave' psycho-therapies, e.g. acceptance and commitment therapy (ACT) and dialectical behavioural therapy (DBT).

DBT was developed by Marsha Linehan, an American psychologist, for the treatment of borderline personality disorder (BPD/EUPD).

Core themes:

- Acceptance of the person as they are, with recognition there is a need to make changes.
- Identifying that 'problem behaviours' (e.g. self-harm or substance use), developed as coping mechanisms for difficult situations, while providing temporary relief, are not effective long-term solutions.
- Assumes that people are doing the best they can but that they need to be supported in learning new, more adaptive ways of coping.
- Incorporates many elements of CBT.
- Includes individual and group sessions (education sessions rather than group therapy).
- Lasts 24 weeks but often repeated up to a year.

Components include:

- Skills' training (mindfulness, distress tolerance, interpersonal effectiveness)—how to ask for what you want and to say no while maintaining interpersonal relationships.
- Emotional regulation (how to be more aware of, and more in control of, emotions).
- Focus on enhancing motivation and ensuring generalization of skills, but within clear, supported boundaries. For example, the person can call for help but can only call between certain hours or they must have tried to implement the skills themselves first.
- Recognizes the need for supporting therapists in delivering this challenging intervention.

16.8.6 Duration of treatment

For acute, discrete presentations (such as acute depression), shorter-term psycho-therapies are used, often using CBT principles. (Although the definition of 'short-term' varies considerably, it would generally be less than a year.) For more enduring problems, particularly enduring issues, such as emotionally unstable personality disorder, psychological interventions are likely to take place over years.

16.9 Summary

The importance of the MDT, a psychological perspective (and intervention) cannot be over-emphasized. As with medical treatments, no single therapy 'cures' all—matching of the psychological intervention with the presenting problems is crucial. An understanding of the development of psychological therapies from psycho-dynamic, through behavioural, cognitive, and more recent interventions, allows the tailoring of psychological interventions to match needs. These may be prescribed on their own or in combination with medical treatments, depending on the nature and severity of the presenting complaint. There are agreed guidelines on the best practice approach to treatment (NICE guidelines (UK) and the Cochrane Database (available online)).

CHAPTER 17

Physical treatments

What you should know about physical treatments in mental health

- How to maximize patient engagement in treatment.
- What are psychotropics.
- Uses and side-effects of anti-depressants and antipsychotics.
- What are mood stabilizers and when are they used.
- Prescribing for anxiety and sleep disorders.
- Physical parameters that must be monitored on antipsychotics.
- ECT—indications and modes of action.

17.1 Introduction

This chapter focuses on physical treatments (medication and ECT). It is not exhaustive, but provides a basic introduction. There are agreed guidelines on the best practice approach to treatment. Useful resources include the NICE guidelines (UK), the Cochrane Database (both available online), and the Maudsley Prescribing Guidelines. It is highly unlikely that you will remember all the side-effects, interactions, and dosage regimens of every medication. If you are not familiar with a drug, **always** check facts before prescribing. Most hospitals now provide an up-to-date formulary on their website.

17.2 Biological treatment: general concepts

Before starting any medication, it is important to have a clear discussion with the patient to ensure that they can make an informed decision about treatment. Many patients do not take their medication as prescribed. There is **no point** in prescribing a medication if the patient is not going to take it.

Discussion with the patient should include:

- Their diagnosis (and reasons why this diagnosis was made).
- Type and name of medication.
- Expected benefits.
- Time to onset of action.
- Likely duration of treatment (if known).
- When and how often to take the medication.
- Need for titration.

- Potential side-effects (starting with the most common).
- Any noteworthy interactions/other medications they should avoid.

Discussion with yourself should include:

- A careful consideration of risks and benefits for the individual; particularly relevant in a hospital setting where patients often have multiple co-morbidities and are on multiple other drugs.
- The old adage 'go low, go slow, and go on' is still relevant today. So start low. Equally, however, there is no point in prescribing sub-therapeutic doses. Gradually titrate the dose (within guidelines) according to response, 'go slow and go on'. It is important that patients are aware that this is your strategy so that they do not become frustrated by a slow rise in improvement. Clearly, there will be situations (see Chapter 18) where rapid, high-dose intervention is needed. As always, intervention must be tailored to the situation.
- Finally, patients should be aware that a drug should not be considered 'ineffective' until it has been taken at an adequate dose for an adequate time (a therapeutic trial) (see Figure 17.1).

Discussions about medication are particularly important for women of **child-bearing age** with a thorough discussion about risks/benefits of treatment versus

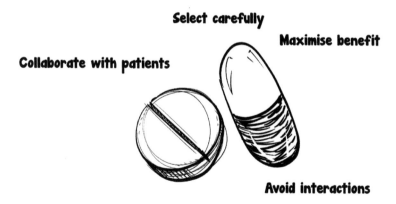

Figure 17.1 Key points to consider when prescribing.
© Eoin Kelleher

no treatment, potential for teratogenicity. Recommendations given to a patient regarding contraception should be clearly documented in their notes. As discussed in Chapter 4, it is important to have **baseline physical parameters** in all patients before starting medication. Finally, it is impossible to remember every drug interaction. Always seek help if unsure (see Practical tips Psychotropic medications)

17.3 What are psychotropics?

Psychotropics are any medications whose main target (and effect), is on mental state (see Table 17.1). Some of the drugs are still called by their older names, e.g. antipsychotics called 'major tranquillizers'/'neuroleptics'. In addition to psychotropics, psychiatrists use two other groups of drugs: anti-epileptic drugs (used in mood disorders) and drugs normally used in Parkinsonism (used to counteract effects of some of the psychotropics). This chapter will present the broad groups of medications, their uses and side-effects. Specific details with respect to individual disorders will be found in the relevant clinical chapters. Cognitive enhancers and psychostimulants are discussed in Chapters 11 and 12, respectively.

Table 17.1 Psychotropics—common medications used in mental illness and their uses

Type	Uses	Examples
Anti-depressants	Depression Anxiety (some) Obsessive–compulsive disorder (some—5HT action)	SSRIs, SNRIs, MAOIs, RIMAs TCADs, NaSSA, MaSSA*
Anxiolytics	Anxiety disorders	Benzodiazepines
Hypnotics	Insomnia	Benzodiazepines and "Z" drugs
Mood stabilizers	Prevention of recurrent mood disorder Augmentation (depression)	Lithium, valproate, carbamazepine, lamotrigine
Antipsychotics	Psychosis Mania Agitation (depression)	First generation Second generation

*SSRI—serotonin specific reuptake inhibitor, SNRI—serotonin noradrenergic reuptake inhibitor, MAOI—monoamine oxidase inhibitor, RIMA (reversible MAOI), TCAs—tricyclic anti-depressants, NaSSA noradrenergic and specific serotonergic anti-depressant, MaSSA—melatonin agonist and specific serotonin antagonist.

17.4 Prescribing in mood disorders

17.4.1 Anti-depressant medication

The most commonly used medications in the treatment of depression are anti-depressants (also useful in anxiety disorders).

In addition to the principles of educating patients generally, it is important that patients are specficially aware that, with anti-depressants:

- While improvement can begin within 10–14 days, it can take up to 6 weeks.
- Usually, an early response predicts a good response.
- Medication should be stopped with medical advice and gradually withdrawn.
- Anti-depressants, like many psychotropics, can be associated with discontinuation symptoms.
- Patients should be seen within 1–2 weeks of starting an anti-depressant to monitor response and side-effects. In particular, patients should be advised about paradoxical effects, such as initial (transient) worsening of agitation, which may require them to stop the medication.

17.4.1.1 Specific anti-depressants

Most anti-depressants affect the monoamines, mainly serotonin (5 hydroxy-tryptamine, 5HT) or noradrenaline, either by directly increasing their availability or via an action on the receptors. Whether this is responsible for their clinical effect has not yet been clearly proven. The choice of anti-depressant is influenced by its:

- Side-effects.
- Drug interactions.
- Therapeutic effects (e.g. mirtazapine associated with sedation, used when insomnia problematic).
- Toxicity in overdose.

As a student or doctor prescribing in a medical setting, SSRIs are the drugs you are most likely to encounter or prescribe. However, other groups, particularly the MAOIs (monoamine oxidase inhibitors) and the TCAs (tricyclic anti-depressants), present particular hazards in a medical setting (see Table 17.2). In all cases, consideration of possible drug–drug interaction is important. If you are not sure, consult your hospital formulary (see Clinical vignette Anti-depressants). Most of the 'newer' anti-depressants are compared to the TCAs, which were, for a long time, the 'gold standard' of anti-depressants.

Table 17.2 Features of main classes of anti-depressants

Type	SSRIs	SNRIs	MAOIs	TCAs
Action	Inhibit reuptake 5HT into presynaptic cell	Inhibit reuptake both 5HT and NorAd	Inhibit MAO (irreversibly)	Increase 5HT, noradrenaline, block acetyl chlorine
Benefits (and compared to TCAs)	Well tolerated Less interactions Safer in OD	Well tolerated Less interactions Safer in OD	Effective but dangerous interactions	Effective but side effects and dangerous in OD
Side-effects	GI (Nausea, Diarrhoea), CNS (Headache, agitation, tremor) Sexual (↓libido, ↓ejaculation) Prolonged QTc, ↓Na⁺ Serotonin syndrome*	GI (Nausea, Diarrhoea), CNS (Headache, agitation, tremor) Sexual (↓libido, ↓ejaculation) Dry mouth Dizziness	Autonomic (dry mouth, constipation, urinary retention, postural bp) CNS (Headache, tremor)	Antichol (dry mouth, constipation, blurred vision, glaucoma, urinary retention) Anti-adrenergic (postural ↓bp) CVS (HR, BP, arrhythmias)
Special considerations	Can worsen agitation initially First-line agents	Possibly more rapid onset "Activating" Discontinuation symptoms Monitor BP at higher doses	Dangerous interactions* (↑bp) with: tyramine foods, drugs that promote 5HT *due to irreversible inhibition of MAO metabolism of other drugs eg opiates, insulin Specialist Rx	Dangerous in OD Seizures
Other uses	Anxiety, OCD		Anxiety (phobia)	Anxiety, OCD (Clomipramine)
Examples	Sertraline, fluoxetine, escitalopram	Venlafaxine, duloxetine	Phenelzine, tranylcypromine	Amitryptiline (NorAd action) clomipramine (5HT action)
Caution or avoid			Other 5HT-acting or pressor drugs	Glaucoma, hepatic failure, prostatism, epilepsy, pregnancy

* See Chapter 18.

17.4.1.2 Other anti-depressants

17.4.1.2.1 Noradrenergic (alpha 2) and specific serotonergic (5HT2) anti-depressant (NaSSA)

For example mirtazapine:

- Useful anti-depressant—a sedative, so useful when prominent agitation or insomnia as part of depression.
- Weight gain and increased appetite—useful when prominent anorexia or weight loss.
- Can cause agranulocytosis (rare, idiosyncratic).
- Comes in orodispersible form (disintegrates in the mouth, easy to swallow).

17.4.1.2.2 Melatonin agonist and specific serotonin antagonist (MaSSA)—agomelatine

- Novel agent.
- May help promote sleep.

17.4.1.2.3 Reversible MAO inhibitors (RIMAs)

- Similar to MAO but reversible inhibition of MAO.
- Reduces risk of hypertensive crises, but still require careful attention to diet.
- Specialist prescriber.

17.4.1.2.4 Modified TCAs

- Lofepramine—tetracyclic, better tolerated than TCAs but can worsen anxiety and insomnia. Less cardiotoxic.
- Trazadone—a sedative, useful to help sleep.

Clinical vignette Anti-depressants

'A 23-year-old university student, referred by her haematologist for assessment, 18 months post-bone marrow transplant, felt she was "just not right". She felt low, disinterested, unable to motivate herself, not enjoying anything she did. While hopeful for the future, she was becoming increasingly despondent. She had tried hard to motivate herself, sticking to a daily routine that included regular exercise and study. She had also read several self-help manuals, trying to implement behavioural and cognitive strategies but still felt "stuck". She had little interest in food, eating only to maintain weight. Her sleep was poor, with difficulty getting off to sleep and broken sleep throughout the night. While she interacted well at interview, engaging and appropriate, she acknowledged this

continued >

---

was not her baseline, and intermittently was tearful and distressed. Collateral history confirmed that she seemed depressed. She had no history of depression and had functioned well. She was very anxious to improve as she was due to return to university.

'Her presentation suggested a depressive episode moderately severe and pervasive. She had already tried many of the early interventions of a psychological approach and lived some distance away, so we agreed a trial of sertraline, an SSRI, starting at a low dose and titrating to 150 mg daily. She tolerated the treatment well and had an excellent response, describing herself as "10/10", back to her baseline within 6 weeks of treatment.

'One of the fascinating things about being a psychiatrist is the similar responses one sees to differing interventions: psychological (e.g. CBT) or medication (e.g. sertraline). This lady returned to university and sport, and excelled at both. She discontinued sertraline, slowly after 6 months and has been discharged from the service.' Liaison Psychiatrist

17.4.2 Mood stabilizers

17.4.2.1 Lithium (Li)

Lithium (a salt) is highly effective in the management of bipolar affective disorder. Its main role is in the prevention of further episodes, particularly mania (mood stabilizer). It also has a role in the management of an acute manic episode. Its mode of action is unknown. It is an effective and widely-used drug but has many side-effects and interactions (see Table 17.3), augmented by its:

- Narrow therapeutic range (0.6–1.0 mmol/l).
- Mode of excretion—it is filtered and partly reabsorbed in the proximal tubules of the kidney with sodium. Any drug which causes dehydration or reduced sodium (e.g. thiazides) will lead to increased reabsorption of lithium and potential toxicity.
- Effect on magnesium and calcium transport leading to interactions with angiotensin converting enzyme (ACE) inhibitors, calcium channel-blockers.

It is a treatment you are likely to encounter within a medical setting and it is important, therefore, that you are aware of these and their management.

Lithium crosses the placenta. A number of **teratogenic effects**, including Epstein's anomaly, floppy baby syndrome, and thyroid abnormalities have been described. It is also secreted into breast milk.

17.4.2.1.1 Schedule for lithium initiation and monitoring

Because of the dangers of lithium toxicity, there is a **specific schedule** for starting and monitoring lithium therapy (please see NICE guidelines). Patients must be well educated about lithium, side-effects, and interactions (see Table 17.3).

Table 17.3 Lithium—side-effects (SE), toxicity and interactions

Early, common SE	Later SE	Li toxicity	Interactions
Polyuria	Polyuria	Nausea, Vomiting	↑Plasma concentration ACE inhibitors, NSAIDs, SSRIs, Ca channel-blockers
Polydyspia	Polydypsia	Coarse Tremor	↑EPSE antipsychotics
Tremor	Hypothyroidism	Confusion*, myoclonic jerks	Impaired glucose tolerance Diabetic medication
Metallic taste	Weight gain	Ataxia, dysarthria, drowsiness	Augments muscle relaxant effect anaesthesia
	Renal impairment Up to 20% renal pathology (e.g. fibrosis) ↓GFR, ↓concentrating ability	Seizures Stupor, Coma Renal and CVS failure	5HT syndrome SSRIs
	Teratogenicity and Breast Feeding implications	*may persist for several weeks	

Baseline checks:

- Physical exam to include BMI and ECG.
- FBC.
- Renal profile to include eGFR.
- TFTs.
- Pregnancy test if indicated.
- Note all other medication.

Lithium—starting and maintenance schedule:

- Starting dose 400–600 mg nocte, increased weekly based on serum monitoring.
- Usual dose 800–1.2 mg daily.

- Monitoring of serum lithium level 7 days after starting and 7 days after each change in dose (blood samples must be taken 12 h post-dose), every 3–6 months once stable.
- Therapeutic level usually 0.6–0.8 mmol/l. Can be maintained at 0.8–1.0 mmol/l in certain circumstances (e.g. resistant disease) but requires specialist input.
- Once established:
  o Monitor weight.
  o Check for side-effects (susceptibility to the effects of lithium appears to increase with age).
  o Lithium level/eGFR every 3 months.
  o TFTs every 6 months.
- If discontinuing treatment, withdraw slowly due to risk of manic relapse.
- Monitor for any new drugs added to treatment.

17.4.2.1.2 Lithium toxicity
Lithium toxicity is a potentially **life-threatening** situation (see Chapter 18).

17.4.2.2 Sodium valproate

- Anti-epileptic, in mental health mainly used as a mood stabilizer (particularly if lithium not tolerated or in rapid cycling disorder).
- Also used in acute manic episode and depression in bipolar affective disorder.
- Plasma levels not used as relationship between serum levels and therapeutic effect unclear (generally use schedule for anti-epileptic effect).
- Dose-dependent teratogenicity—avoid in women of child-bearing age unless under expert care.
- Side-effects include:
  o Nausea, vomiting.
  o Sedation.
  o Blood dyscrasias.
  o Raised liver enzymes, hepatotoxicity.
  o Rare, but dangerous, adverse effects, e.g. irreversible liver failure and pancreatitis.
- Interactions with lamotrigine (inhibits metabolism) and other high protein-bound drugs.

17.4.2.3 Carbamazepine

- Anti-epileptic, used in mental health in bipolar affective disorder (second line agent).

- Less effective than lithium.
- Used in:
  - O Prophylaxis in bipolar affective disorder.
  - O Acute mania.
  - O Acute depressive episode.
- Side-effects include:
  - O Ataxia, sedation, and dizziness.
  - O Hyponatremia and blood dyscrasias.
  - O Steven–Johnson syndrome.
  - O Acute pancreatitis.
- May be fatal in overdose.
- Plasma levels not generally used; monitor for side-effects.
- Interactions: a potent inducer of cP450 enzyme, so reduces plasma levels of multiple drugs,

17.4.2.4 *Lamotrigine*

- Anti-epileptic, in mental health mainly used as a mood stabilizer (depressive phase).
- Slow introduction and increase in dose.
- Side-effects include:
  - O Nausea, vomiting.
  - O Dizziness, headache, blurred vision.
  - O Rash, which may be severe (toxic epidermal necrolysis).
  - O Blood dyscrasias.
- Interacts with valproate (increased levels), and carbamazepine (neurotoxiity).
- Teratogenesis—cleft palate.

17.4.3 Augmentation (and switching) strategies

Monotherapy, use of a single agent, is best. **Augmentation** is used where there is a partial response to medication. **Switching,** to another agent, is used where there is no response to the first agent. In 'treatment-resistant' depression, anti-depressants may be combined with another agent. Combining medications increases the risk of side-effects. This should be clearly explained to patients before commencing treatment.

Medications used to **augment** treatment with anti-depressants include:

- Mood stabilizers typically used in the treatment of bipolar affective disorders (lithium or lamotrigine).
- Antipsychotic medications, such as quetiapine, that also have an effect on serotonin.

> **Practical tips** Psychotropic medications
>
> It is almost impossible to remember all the side-effects, doses, and interactions.
> You should know general information about prescribing in psychiatry and examples of each of the classes of drugs, e.g. antipsychotics, anti-depressants, mood stabilizers, etc.
> For students who work outside psychiatry but encounter patients on psychotropic medications within a medical setting, what is particularly important is:
> • You identify their history and medications by taking a careful history.
> • You seek information from their psychiatrist and GP.
> • You ensure their medication is correctly prescribed.
> • You are alert to drugs that pose particular risks, e.g. lithium, clozapine, MAOIs; side-effects/interactions that pose particular risks, e.g. prolonged QTc (antipsychotics), serotonin syndrome (SSRIs).
> • You ask for help/check with the hospital pharmacist or prescriber if you have any concerns.

17.4.4 Electro-convulsive therapy (ECT)

This is used in specialist situations only. Its indications include:

• Treatment-resistant depression (less commonly, mania, psychosis).
• Catatonia (schizophrenia, depression).
• Urgent, rapid intervention, e.g. severe depression where patient refuses all intake, puerperal psychosis,

The mechanism of action remains unknown but seems to depend on the brain response (seizure activity) not on the motor response. It requires, therefore, a (brief) anaesthetic and neuromuscular paralysis while an electric current is applied via an electrode placed either on each side of the head (bilateral ECT) or one side (unilateral). Unilateral placement on the non-dominant side at high dose seems as effective as bilateral but with less cognitive side-effects. Theories of action include neurochemical, neuroendocrine, and sleep disruption processes. Its main benefit is in rapidity of response and response in specific situations as previously discussed. As the intervention requires an anaesthetic, there is a strict protocol of work-up prior to ECT, including liaison with the anaesthetist.

17.5 Anxiolytics/hypnotics prescribing in anxiety disorders

• The management of anxiety disorders starts, as with all disorders, with a careful assessment ensuring the correct diagnosis and formulation. Because physical symptoms abound in anxiety disorders it is particularly important to exclude physical illness (see Chapter 8).

- Psychological interventions, particularly CBT, are often more appropriate.
- Because they are highly addictive and rarely treat the underlying condition, simply 'dampening' symptoms of anxiety, they should be prescribed sparingly. Anxiolytics are best limited to brief periods, often in the context of overwhelming distress, while other interventions are started. The most widely used anxiolytics are the benzodiazepines.

17.5.1 Benzodiazepines (BDZ)

- BDZs are anxiolytic, sedative, used as hypnotics. They increase the seizure threshold and act as muscle relaxants. They bind to the BDZ receptor site on the $GABA_A$ receptor. The choice of BDZ depends on the underlying problem and is usually based on length of action:
  - ○ Short-acting (oxazepam, lorazepam) when rapid onset, short-lived action is required (e.g. rapid tranquillization, anticipatory nausea) or as a hypnotic (e.g. temazepam) to avoid hang-over effects the next day.
  - ○ Longer acting agents (e.g. chlordiazepoxide, diazepam) used in chronic anxiety or in withdrawal where you want to ensure the effects do not wear off.
- While BDZs are generally well-tolerated (initially) with minimal drug interactions, they are strongly associated with dependence and, particularly in the elderly, are associated with an increased risk of falls and confusion. Other possible side-effects include sedation, impaired performance (driving, operating machinery), and headache. Paradoxical inhibition (aggravation/release of aggressive or impulsive behaviours) with BDZs is often cited in textbooks. The effects of BDZs can be reversed acutely with flumazenil, a BDZ receptor antagonist, if needed, rarely, in severe BDZ overdose. Please be aware that, if the patient has taken a long-acting BDZ in overdose (OD), the effects of the flumazenil will wear off more quickly than the BDZ, so on-going monitoring will be required.
- **Withdrawal effects**, common on stopping BDZs, particularly if used for several months, are an **important presentation**, particularly on in-patient wards (see Chapter 10).

17.5.2 Beta-blockers

These drugs mask the physical symptoms of anxiety (tachycardia, tremor). However, as they do not treat the underlying disorder and are themselves associated with significant side-effects (e.g. bradycardia, bronchospasm), a purist approach would suggest they only be used if absolutely necessary.

17.5.3 Buspirone

Buspirone is a 5HT1a agonist that has anxiolytic properties. It does not act at the GABA receptor and is not associated with the tolerance and dependence of BDZs. It has some efficacy in the treatment of generalised anxiety disorder. Side-effects include headache and nausea.

17.5.4 Anti-depressants

If pharmacotherapy is required for the treatment of anxiety disorders (severe anxiety disorder, unresponsive to, or unsuitable for, psychotherapy), anti-depressants are the most appropriate choice. The SSRIs are most commonly used given their relative safety in overdose and their favourable side-effect profile. However, please note that symptoms are generally slower to respond than mood symptoms (up to 8 weeks for full response) and some drugs may initially cause a mild increase in anxiety and agitation (start at a low dose and advise the patient). **Mirtazapine**, which reduces anxiety and can help with insomnia and anorexia, is another option.

17.5.5 Prescribing for insomnia (hypnotics)

Generally, it is wise to avoid prescribing medication for sleep disturbance, try instead to understand the reason for the insomnia and treat the underlying causes. This may include intervention for a major mental illness causing insomnia (e.g. major depression or mania), pain, environmental or lifestyle factors that are disrupting the sleep cycle. Advice and education about good 'sleep hygiene' is then the mainstay of treatment. Any hypnotic will invariably disrupt the underlying sleep cycle and is potentially addictive, so should only be prescribed in the lowest dose possible for the shortest time possible and where clinically indicated.

Short-acting benzodiazepines (e.g. temazepam) and the newer non-benzodiazepine drugs (zolpidem and zopiclone, so-called 'Z-drugs') are most commonly prescribed. Both classes work by potentiating GABA activity. Z-drugs have a different structure to the benzodiazepines and were thought to be less likely to induce dependence and have a quicker onset of action and elimination. However, both classes are associated with significant risks and, especially in the elderly, are associated with increased risk of falls and impaired balance and decision-making. Risks of abuse and tolerance are higher with the benzodiazepine drugs.

17.6 Prescribing in psychotic disorders

17.6.1 Antipsychotic medication

An antipsychotic (also called a neuroleptic) is a drug used to:

- Treat the acute symptoms of psychosis (hallucinations, delusions, agitation).
- Prevent relapse of psychosis.
- Reduce psychomotor agitation (in the context of mania or organic brain syndromes).

Many of the antipsychotics achieve this without significant sedation. Antipsychotics are the mainstay of treatment in **psychotic disorders** (see Chapter 7). They are also used as additional treatment in mood disorders (see Chapter 6), particularly in BPAD where they are used both in maintenance treatment and in the management of acute episodes.

The **first-generation** (older, 'typical') antipsychotics (FGAs) primarily block D2 receptors, although they also affect alpha-adrenergic, histaminergic, and muscarinic receptors. The D2 blockade is thought to be responsible for treating 'positive' symptoms of psychosis (hallucinations and delusions). It is also responsible for most extra-pyramidal side-effects (EPSEs) (see Table 17.4). The newer, '**second-generation**' (SGA) antipsychotics (also termed 'atypical' due to their less prominent EPSEs and different receptor profile) block serotonergic (5HT2) receptors to varying degrees, in addition to varying effects at the D2 receptor. The second-generation antipsychotics had been viewed as being more efficacious than the first generation, but, apart from clozapine in treatment-resistant schizophrenia, this has, more recently, been called into question. Most of the differences lie in their side-effect profile (see Tables 17.4, 17.5).

If patients fail to respond to a therapeutic trial of at least 2 different antipsychotic drugs (one of which must have been an SGA, this is termed '**treatment-resistant schizophrenia**' and **clozapine** should be offered (Chapter 17).

For the older, 'typical', '**first generation**' antipsychotics (FGA), the main **mode of action,** is blockade of dopamine (DA) receptors (specifically the D2 receptor), although they also have varying effects on alpha-adrenergic, histaminergic and muscarinic receptors

17.6.2 Metabolic syndrome

This term is used to describe slightly differing syndromes, although all associated with an increased risk of diabetes. In the context of schizophrenia, key items include:

- Insulin resistance with raised fasting glucose.
- Increased fat deposition (especially abdominal).
- Abnormal lipid profile (increased triglycerides, reduce HDL).

It is associated with an increased risk of:

- Type 2 diabetes.
- Cardiovascular disease (stroke, ischaemic heart disease).

Abnormal inflammatory markers (C-reactive protein (CRP), tumour necrosis factor (TNF)) may also be present. Patients with schizophrenia have a significantly increased risk of diabetes. This is greater with SGAs than with FGAs but has been found in patients with schizophrenia independent of drug use. Careful monitoring of all parameters (see Table 17.6), advice on lifestyle for weight control, or switching antipsychotic may be necessary

Table 17.4 Main side-effects antipsychotics

Extra-pyramidal (ESPEs)	Anti-cholinergic	Anti-adrenergic
Acute dystonia Painful contraction muscle group young males, esp. head/neck, (acute torticollis), eyes (oculogyric crisis), Onset early (hours) Rx anticholinergic, switch to less potent drug	Dry mouth, blurred vision, worsening glaucoma Urinary retention Constipation	Postural hypotension Delayed ejaculation
Parkinsonism Ridigity, bradykinesia, tremor, Onset days to weeks Rx reduce dose, switch, or add anti-cholinergic	Arrythmias Prolonged QTc	Neuroleptic malignant syndrome (see Chapter 18, Emergencies)
Akathisia Distressing sense of restlessness, cannot sit still, difficult to distinguish from agitation, Onset hours to weeks Rx switch, add B blocker	**Weight Gain** Particularly with olanzapine, clozapine, phenothiazines Mechanism unclear	**Anti-histaminergic** Sedation
Tardive dyskinesia Slow, writhing movements, especially lips/tongue (chewing sucking), Onset months, years Often unaware Often irreversible Reduction in dose, anticholinergics may worsen Rx Tetrabenzaine, switch to clozapine	**Hyperprolactinaemia** Galactorrhoea, Amenorrhea, Gyaecomastia Hypogonadism Osteoporosis	**Dyslipidaemia** inc TGs and cholesterol
Tardive dystonia/akathisia Late presentation of above syndromes Difficult to treat	**Blood dyscrasias** Especially clozapine (agranulocytosis) (Care post bone marrow suppression)	

Table 17.5 Differing antipsychotic side-effect profiles (simplified version)

Type	'Typical' FGAs	'Atypical' SGAs
Example	Haloperidol, chlorpromazine, trifluoperazine, fluphenazine	Risperidone, olanzapine, clozapine, quetiapine, aripiprazole, paliperidone
EPSEs	Frequent	Infrequent
Anticholinergic	Frequent	Infrequent except clozapine
Antiadrenergic	Frequent	Infrequent
Anti-histaminergic	Frequent	Infrequent except clozapine
Hyperprolactinaemia	Frequent	Infrequent except risperidone
Arrythmias Prolonged QTc	Frequent	Frequent except aripiprazole
Weight gain	Frequent except haloperidol	Frequent (especially olanzapine, clozapine) Infrequent aripiprazole
Metabolic syndrome (dyslipidaemia, glucose intolerance)	Infrequent	Frequent especially clozapine, olanzapine

17.6.3 Practicalities of prescribing

Baseline investigations before starting antipsychotics should include weight, waist circumference, pulse/BP, fasting blood sugar/HbA1c, and baseline nutritional and physical activity status, and baseline ECG and repeated throughout treatment (see Table 17.6).

As always, **start with a low dose** and slowly titrate upwards, depending on clinical response.

Education about the drug, side effects, and the risk of co-morbid substance abuse should be given.

17.6.4 Which antipsychotic to use?

The choice of agent will be influenced by:

- Presenting features.
- Balance between benefits and side-effects:
  o Metabolic—weight gain/diabetes.
  o Extrapyramidal—akathisia/dyskinesia.
  o Cardiovascular—prolonged QT interval on the ECG.
- Patients' views.

Table 17.6 Monitoring of physical parameters on antipsychotics

	Baseline	Month 1	Month 2	Month 3	Month 6	Subsequent
BMI	x	x	x	x	x	3 monthly
Waist	x	x	x	x	x	3 monthly
BP	x			x	x	3 monthly
Fasting glucose	x			x	x	3 monthly
Fasting lipids	x				x	Annually

Thus, for example, if sedation is needed, FGA may be useful. If there is a significant mood component, quetiapine or olanzapine may be indicated (see Table 17.5). Generally, SGAs are now used as first-line in newly diagnosed schizophrenia. Profile and bioavailability of the drug will also be relevant.

- **Haloperidol**: potent DA blockade, available in oral, IM and IV (rarely used) preparations, useful in rapid tranquillization.
- **Olanzapine**: available in oro-dispersible form, sedating, useful in agitated patients.
- **Risperidone**: less sedative, minimal extra-pyramidal side-effects.
- **Fluphenazine**: poor compliance, **depot** medication.
- **Clozapine**: failure to respond to adequate trials of at least two anti-psychotics (one of which is FGA).

17.6.5 Clozapine: special considerations

Clozapine was the first SGA and remains a pivotal drug in this group due to its particular effectiveness in treatment-resistant schizophrenia (see Clinical vignette Clozapine). Initially withdrawn from use due to fatal agranulocytosis, it has since been re-introduced but requires careful monitoring. Like lithium, because of its side-effects and the critical protocols for its use, you are likely to encounter it in medical practice and so need to be aware of the guidelines for its use. The list below is not exhaustive (refer to NICE guidelines/BNF if needed):

- Used in schizophrenia unresponsive to an adequate trial of at least two antipsychotics.
- Reduces rate of suicide in schizophrenia.
- Action on D1, D4 receptors, less effect on D2 (thus relatively fewer EPSEs).
- Significant anti-cholinergic, histaminergic, and adrenergic effects (see Tables 17.4, 17.5), including hypersalivation and constipation.

- Rare, but potentially life-threatening side effects:
  - Fatal agranulocytosis, thrombocytopenia, myocarditis, nephritis.
  - Acute organic brain state.
  - Seizures (dose-related).
  - Risk of respiratory depression when combined with BDZs.
- Dosing schedule:
  - Patient must be registered with a clozapine monitoring service (CPMS in Ireland and the UK).
  - In addition to usual baseline tests, a confirmed normal white cell (neutrophil) count must be confirmed pre-treatment.
  - Weekly FBCs for first 18 weeks, fortnightly for a year, then monthly thereafter for as long as the patient is taking the medication.
  - Slow gradual titration of dose, starting at 12.5 mg day 1, 25 mg day 2 then increases of 25–50 mg daily (each escalation over 14–21 days).
  - Usual dose 450 mg daily, risk of seizures above 600 mg/day.
  - CPMS employs a 'traffic light' system with regard to WCC/neutrophil levels:
    - Red: stop immediately, monitor FBC, get haematology advice, avoid other antipsychotics.
    - Amber: proceed with caution, monitor neutrophils daily with CPMS advice.
    - Green: proceed.
- Variation in clozapine levels and particular relevance in medical hospitals:
  - As clozapine undergoes extensive first-pass metabolism in the liver, it is particularly susceptible to drug interactions.
  - Sudden cessation of smoking (e.g. hospital admission) can increase plasma levels.
  - Sudden discontinuation (e.g. hospital admission) is not advised due to risk of cholinergic rebound with sweating, headache, nausea, and vomiting.
  - If clozapine is stopped for more than 48 h, it must be re-introduced slowly following the aforementioned protocol above.

Clinical vignette Clozapine

'I have never forgotten a case, as a surgical trainee, of a 45-year-old man who was admitted with an acute abdomen requiring emergency surgery. He had been acutely unwell and confused on presentation to the ED and was rapidly transferred for surgery. In the post-operative period, while recovering well from his surgery, he became increasingly agitated, irritable, and suspicious of staff. Initially, this was felt to be delirium, as he had developed a pyrexia and chest infection. However, on review of his case, it was noted he had a history of schizophrenia, stable for many years on clozapine (450 mg daily), which had not been prescribed since admission. Collateral history from his mental health team revealed he had treatment-resistant schizophrenia, responding only to clozapine

continued >

and when psychotic previously had become severely paranoid, aggressive, and challenging to manage. As he had now been off clozapine for more than 48 h, the drug had to be re-introduced slowly, starting at 12.5 mg daily as per the clozapine protocol. Management of his paranoid psychosis and associated behavioural disturbance in the intervening period, while titrating up his clozapine, was very challenging. I have never forgotten to check for mental health history and medication since then.' Consultant Surgeon

17.6.6 Depot medication

Some patients find it difficult to take oral medication. Antipsychotics can be given in long-acting form (a 'depot'—the active drug is in an oily suspension) by intramuscular injection (usually gluteal muscle but some can be given in the deltoid). Patients must be administered a 'test dose' to ensure they can tolerate the drug. Issues include the need for careful titration of the dose, an awareness that the drug will remain in the system for longer than an oral formulation (meaning any adverse effects will take longer to resolve) and pain/discomfort at the injection site. **It is important to ensure patients admitted to a medical hospital continue to receive their depot, if prescribed.**

17.6.7 Prescribing in specific situations

It is not possible to remember the settings for metabolism of all drugs. Renal, hepatic, or cardiac impairment can all affect drug clearance, metabolism, and toxicity, so it is essential to check the drug's information sheet and advice regarding prescribing in special situations. Some drugs will be contra-indicated in specific situations, e.g. clozapine in severe renal impairment.

17.6.7.1 Renal impairment

Any drug cleared predominantly by the kidney will naturally accumulate in the presence of renal impairment, with risks of higher serum levels and dose-related side-effects. General advice in the presence of renal impairment is to start at lower doses, increase slowly, and monitor for side-effects. If patients are on dialysis, liaise with the patient's renal physician. In all cases, check the drugs profile and side-effects for specific advice in the presence of renal impairment.

17.6.7.2 Liver impairment

Most psychotropics are metabolized by the liver. Most levels will be increased in the presence of liver disease and will require lower initial starting doses. In more severe liver disease, be aware of the possibility of precipitating hepatic encephalopathy with sedative drugs, such as benzodiazepines.

17.6.7.3 Cardiovascular disease (CVD)

QTc prolongation increases the risk of fatal arrhythmias and is potentiated by several psychotropics, including antipsychotics (particularly the phenothiazines)

and anti-depressants (TCAs and citalopram). A baseline ECG should be done prior to starting medication and the presence of cardiac disease, such as myocardial ischaemia, myocarditis, or other medications that affect cardiac conduction, must be noted.

Drugs such as phenothiazines and clozapine may cause hypotension and/or tachycardia; high-dose venlafaxine is associated with hypertension.

17.6.7.4 Epilepsy

Many psychotropics lower the seizure threshold. This is generally a dose-related phenomenon, so starting at a low dose and careful titration is essential. The SSRIs (for depression) and haloperidol (as an antipsychotic) are the most appropriate in the presence of epilepsy. Awareness of possible interaction with anti-epileptic medication is also important. At high doses, clozapine may cause seizures. This is likely to require dose reduction, and/or addition of an anti–epilepsy agent, such as valproate.

17.6.7.5 Pregnancy

Please see Chapter 12.

17.7 Summary

A range of presentations in mental health will require psychotropic medication. It is important to be aware of the main classes of drugs, the indications for their use, their side-effects, and interactions. Any presentation will be influenced by psychological and social factors, as well as biological ones, and interventions must reflect that.

CHAPTER 18

Emergencies: urgent, serious, and high-risk scenarios in psychiatry

CHAPTER FOCUS

What you should know about emergencies in psychiatry
- How to manage **acute behavioural disturbance**.
- How to assess 'risk', including harm to self and others.
- How to recognize and manage other emergencies that commonly occur in a medical setting including:
  - Neuroleptic malignant syndrome.
  - Serotonin syndrome.
  - Lithium toxicity.

18.1 Introduction

The term 'emergency' causes many people to freeze, gripped by panic, rendering them unable to have a clear plan of action. This is particularly likely for inexperienced, newly qualified doctors. Examples of urgent, serious, high-risk scenarios in psychiatry (particularly those likely to present in medical settings) include acute behavioural disturbance, risk of harm to self or others, neuroleptic malignant syndrome, serotonin syndrome, and lithium toxicity. This is not an exhaustive list. Discussion on some 'emergencies' is already embedded in the chapters on the illnesses with which they present.

In **every** interaction with our patients we need to consider risk and safety. If we conduct every interview as if there is potential risk to self or others, we will not be seen to be 'judging' or 'stigmatizing' certain patients. Furthermore, we will be prepared (as much as is possible) for the unexpected. Similarly, for medication-related 'emergencies', careful attention to every prescription, (drug interactions, side-effects), is crucial. Emergencies should not be seen in isolation. Nonetheless, there will always be scenarios where one is called to an 'emergency' and this chapter highlights some of these.

18.2 Acute behavioural disturbance

Clinical vignette Acute behavioural disturbance

'I will never forget my first night on-call as a psychiatry trainee in a large psychiatry unit in inner-city London. Within the first hour of taking the bleep, I was called urgently to the Emergency Department where four staff members were trying to calm and contain an extremely agitated, powerful young man who was shouting and abusive. I could see the nurses and attendants were at risk of injury (as was the man himself, who was shouting, banging his head against the wall). I did not know anything about him—did he have a mental illness? Was he on medication? Did he have any drug allergies? I stood there, frozen, while the experienced nursing staff tried to manage the situation. What to do now?'
Consultant Psychiatrist

It is an irony in medical training that it is often the newest, youngest, most junior trainee who is first called (sometimes by senior doctors and/or nurses in another area) to assess agitated, aggressive, and challenging situations (see Clinical vignette Acute behavioural disturbance). It is also equally disappointing for anyone committed to the care of patients who struggle with their mental health, that these scenarios are so prominent in discussions about mental illness. Very, very few of our patients present in this manner. Very few of our patients are aggressive or violent. However, inevitably, if working in a busy city-centre hospital, one will be called to these situations. Many of these presentations are NOT due to mental illness.

18.2.1 Acute behavioural disturbance: initial response
A clear idea of one's role in these situations is crucial (Figure 18.1):

- First, make the situation as **safe** as possible for everyone, to enable you to make an assessment. This may mean moving other patients away from the environment, or moving the person presenting (if possible) to a quieter (supervised) area on their own. If the person is carrying a weapon (rare), you may need to involve the police.

- Always ensure you have **enough staff** with you to maximize safety. While this hampers the development of rapport, until you are clearer about the situation, putting yourself and others at risk must be avoided or minimized.

- **Even more** than in routine assessment, it is vital to go through the steps of a careful, objective assessment of the situation before rushing in to 'do something'. To corrupt a well-known maxim 'don't just do something, stand there'. The management of acute behavioural disturbance may, to ensure safety, require restraint (an unpleasant experience for all involved)

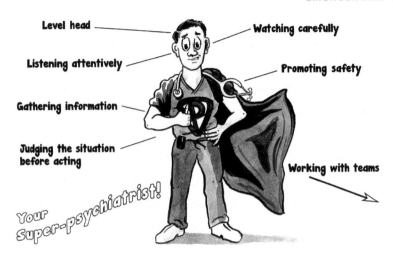

Level head

Listening attentively

Gathering information

Judging the situation
before acting

Watching carefully

Promoting safety

Working with teams

Your Super-psychiatrist!

Figure 18.1 Emergencies—how to be a 'super-psychiatrist'.
© Eoin Kelleher.

and emergency sedation (with the risk of adverse drug reactions), together with resultant difficulty in examining the patient further until the
sedation wears off. It is important to **have as much information as is safely
possible** before intervening.

- A decision as to **whether or not the person is suffering from a mental
illness** is key. There are many reasons for acute behavioural disturbance.
These range from acute organic brain states, intoxication due to substance abuse, to acute psychotic illness. These will require your input and
expertise. In some cases, however, there will be no mental illness. The
person is angry and aggressive for other reasons. It is very important to be
clear in this latter scenario, liaise with medical staff to communicate this to
them, and other interventions (involvement of security or the police) can
then be made, as needed.

The assessment in these scenarios will often have to take place with very little
history available from the patient:

- **Collateral history** is crucial from:
  - Staff in the Emergency Department (ED) with respect to what they know and
    have observed on this presentation or on previous presentations.
  - Relatives (if possible).
  - Other medical staff (GP, community mental health team).

○ The police may have brought in the person and can provide crucial background information.

- Access to medical notes, and ED's notes or letters can transform a very difficult assessment.

○ For example, one may find the person has a history of bipolar affective disorder, recently stopped their medication, and presented similarly 5 years previously, requiring admission under the Mental Health Act. Equally, one may see the patient has a history of acute dystonic reaction to haloperidol with advice to avoid the drug in the future. It is very distressing, for everyone involved, to discover this 5 minutes after one has given an IM dose of haloperidol.

It is crucial, therefore, despite the pressing circumstances, to **gather as much information as possible before acting.**

In the real world of course, as in the Clinical vignette, this is not always possible. The patient is so agitated and behaviourally disturbed, potentially harming themselves or others, that one must move to sedation rapidly. As always, clinical management requires balancing of risks in a real-world scenario. In cases where there is uncertainty, one can, for example, use only a benzodiazepine (which carries the lowest risk of interaction/adverse effects) initially until the situation is clearer

18.2.2 Protocol for acute behavioural disturbance

Almost every hospital now has a (regularly updated) protocol for the management of behavioural disturbance. **Consult your hospital formulary for guidance.** These protocols are only implemented after careful assessment.

The general principles are:

- Make the situation as safe as possible to allow careful assessment.
- First try to engage the person by speaking to them as calmly as possible.
- Move to oral medication, if necessary.
- If this fails, escalate to restraint and sedation in a graduated way (as per hospital guidelines) (NB It can take 20–30 min for medication to take effect, so avoid giving doses in rapid succession).

Figures 18.2 and **18.3** are from the St. James's Hospital (Dublin) formulary and are given to illustrate general concepts only. You must consult an up-to-date protocol from your hospital formulary. There are different guidelines for older adults (smaller doses of medication are advised). The examples given apply to those aged 18 and over.

18.3 Assessment of 'risk'

As discussed in Chapter 15, concepts such as 'risk' and 'risk assessment' are difficult, as they are all attempts to predict the future; in effect, an impossible task.

Patients under 65	Patients 65 and Older
Haloperidol 2.5mg–10mg PO and/or Lorazepam 2mg PO Maximum Haloperidol 20mg/24 hours Maximum Lorazepam 8mg/24 hours	Haloperidol 0.5mg–1mg PO and/or Lorazepam 0.5mg-1 mg PO Aim not more than 2mg Haloperidol in 24 hours (if never on antipsychotic before) Maximum Lorazepam 2mg/24 hours
Olanzapine can be used if Haloperidol is contraindicated Olanzapine 10mg PO Max dose of 20mg/24 hours Lorazepam and Olanzapine together can lead to excessive somnolence	Olanzapine 2.5mg PO Aim for not more than 5mg/24 hours due to risk of side effects **Olanzapine is not licensed for use in BPSD and is associated with an increased risk of stroke in those 65 and older**

Figure 18.2 St. James's Hospital rapid tranquillization protocol—oral medication.
Reproduced courtesy of St James's Hospital.*#
*Ages 18 and over.
#Illustrative only and constantly updated, please refer to your own, up-to-date hospital guidelines.

Nonetheless, we can focus on areas where our input can be helpful. In particular, we can assess risk of harm:

• In a specific situation.
• In a specific context.

The aim is to identify factors (historical, social, clinical) that may be associated with increased risk. In particular, we want to identify factors where we can intervene, e.g. clinical factors, such as an acute psychosis.

In some cases, we can judge the **immediate risk** to be so great that the patient requires admission to hospital. It should be noted, however, that even admission to hospital, often seen as the final great protector, first, does not reduce the risk to zero, and, second, is not without its own adverse outcomes: for the patient admitted, for other patients on the ward (or for other patients for whom scarce resources are now unavailable), or for staff. Real-life scenarios,

Patients under 65

Haloperidol 2.5mg–5mg 1M
and/or
Lorazepam 2mg 1M
Maximum Haloperidol 20mg/24
hours
Maximum Lorazepam 8mg/24 hours

Patients physical obs should be
monitored every 15 minutes for an
hour and every 30 minutes thereafter
until they are mobile

Patients 65 and older

Haloperidol 0.5mg–1mg 1M
and/or
Lorazepam 0.5mg–1mg 1M
Aim for not more than 2mg
Haloperidol in 24 hours (if never on
antipsychotic before)
Maximum Lorazepam 2mg/24 hours

Patients physical obs should be
monitored every 15 minutes for an
hour and every 30 minutes thereafter
until they are mobile

Figure 18.3 St. James's Hospital rapid tranquillization protocol—IM medication.
Reproduced courtesy of St James's Hospital.*#
*Ages 18 and over.
#Illustrative only and constantly updated, please refer to your own, up-to-date hospital guidelines.

as always, are complex. Thus, for example, a patient with repetitive self-harm in the context of borderline personality disorder (a high-risk situation) may be working with their team to build skills in managing distress and move to an independent life without recurrent admissions to hospital—something they can never acquire if they are repeatedly admitted. Other persons seeking admission (who may be engaging in impulsive, high-risk behaviour) may not, as discussed above, have a mental illness and their admission to the ward may be hugely disruptive to other patients. All these situations carry risk, however. The patient with borderline personality disorder and repetitive self-harm runs the risk of dying by suicide, yet, they cannot progress to life outside hospital without running some risk. These are very difficult clinical scenarios, much like in medicine or surgery, where complex decisions must be made (such as balancing the risk of death due to surgery with the risk of death without surgery). We must make them to the absolute best of our ability, in the best interests of our patients, using all the resources available. For junior doctors, asking for help and support from senior colleagues is essential.

18.4 Risk of harm to self

Assessment of risk of self-harm is an intrinsic part of any assessment of mental health. The degree to which it is pursued depends on the circumstances of the presentation. This differs, for example, between someone who has presented having self-harmed and someone presenting with mild anxiety actively seeking help.

First, one needs to be clear about the difference between 'self-harm' and 'attempted suicide'. Broadly speaking, in the former scenario the patient will tell you they did not intend to die, but harmed themselves to relieve distress. Often the method supports this, e.g. superficial cuts to the forearm.

The person who 'attempted suicide' usually says they intended to die, and the method, again, often supports this, e.g. attempted hanging. As always, careful history, collateral history, and examination are essential (see Chapter 2). The information helps to guide decisions about the best management for the individual but, as underlined in the discussion about risk (see Chapter 15), sadly it is impossible to always predict accurately those who will die by suicide. This is particularly the case in the ED where many patients present with self-harm. Our role is to identify any areas in which we can intervene to help. As always, careful assessment helps to guide management.

18.4.1 Factors to consider when assessing presentations with self-harm/attempted suicide

The **literature** provides a list of factors **associated** with suicide. These include:

- Male gender:
  - Women attempt suicide more often than men but men are more likely to complete suicide.
- Single/divorced/widowed.
- Living alone.
- Limited social supports.
- Unemployed or lower socio-economic status.
- Previous history of deliberate self-harm or a previous suicide attempt.
- Diagnosis of a mental disorder.
- Substance use.
- Recent discharge from a psychiatric unit.
- Recent loss or bereavement.
- Co-morbid physical illness.

This list of factors associated with suicide **may not help the clinician in the emergency department** where very many people present with these risk factors—young, male, poor social supports, substance abuse, unemployed, and often significant losses. So, while they are enshrined in the literature, their specificity is poor and positive predictive value low, particularly for clinicians involved in real-life decisions (see Chapter 15). Nonetheless, the information helps to inform assessment and to highlight any areas one can intervene. Ultimately, the aim of a competent risk assessment is to ascertain if:

- There initially was suicidal intent (as this presentation is different from those who wanted to self-harm but not to die).
- There is ongoing suicidal intent.
- There is an underlying mental disorder.
- There are any risk factors that can be modified, and if so, when and how might that best be done.

18.4.1.1 Method of self-harm

Often, the method used will give an indication of the perceived lethality of the event. Thus, a patient who has presented with a self-inflicted shotgun wound, attempted hanging, and jumping in front of a train, or from a height, will always present as high-risk, while cases of overdose or self-cutting may present more complex pictures. With respect to overdose, for example, the substance taken and the number of tablets taken are indicators of apparent lethality.

18.4.1.2 Context of self-harm

The following factors suggest pre-planning and/or active efforts to ensure lethality of the event:

- Ensuring they will not be found/going to a remote place.
- Leaving a note.
- Putting their affairs in order (making a will, giving away a pet).
- Stockpiling medication for the overdose/carefully planned method.

Conversely, for example, an overdose of a small number of tablets that were immediately available, in the presence of others, in the context of a heated argument, suggests an impulsive act.

18.4.1.3 History of mental illness

The rates of suicide are increased in all mental illness—some (e.g. depression, schizophrenia) more than others. Therefore, any history of mental illness significantly increases risk and must be carefully assessed (see Chapter 6).

Certain factors in each illness are worrying findings. Thus, for example, in depression the presence of hopelessness or delusions of guilt would be concerning. In schizophrenia, co-morbid depression or command hallucinations also suggest increased risk of suicide. Recent changes in medication or increased stressful life events also suggest an increased risk and indicate factors that may be modified.

18.4.1.4 Stressors and supports

An assessment of stressors and supports in each case is important. Stresses may include financial, relationship, family, or work issues. Supports include family (partner, children, parents), supportive, structured work environment, or friends.

18.4.1.5 Substance abuse

Assessing deliberate self-harm in the context of substance abuse is an example of the complexity of presentations. Sometimes patients will clearly say they took an 'accidental overdose' in order to 'get a high'. Other patients will only self-harm in the context of alcohol and will bitterly regret the attempt. Others will deliberately get intoxicated as part of a serious attempt on their life. Each of these presentations must be carefully examined to try to fully understand the context of what is happening.

18.4.1.6 Patients' own view

Often patients will be clear themselves about what they have done and whether they intended to die. It is important also to ask their current view now that they have survived, whether they can see a future for themselves now, how they feel about what has happened.

18.4.1.7 Family history of suicide

There is a genetic contribution to suicide but its association is unclear and while this is routinely asked, it will not be particularly helpful in a real-life scenario in the emergency department. Nonetheless, if members of the family have died by suicide, this is an important factor to consider, not only for the (possible) genetic contribution, but also for the distress the family will have suffered.

18.4.1.8 Previous history of self-harm/attempted suicide

It is a fact that previous self-harm is associated with ultimate suicide, confirming the maxim that the only true predictor of future behaviour is previous behaviour. However, because so many people who have self-harmed do **not** die by suicide, this finding is not necessarily helpful in a real-life situation in the ED. Nonetheless, careful history of the circumstances and nature of any previous attempts does inform the current assessment (e.g. violent method, requiring medical admission/ ICU admission/admission to psychiatric unit). Furthermore, a history of recent onset of attempted self-harm, with escalation of episodes in recent weeks is a worrying history.

18.4.1.9 Medication history

A knowledge of the person's current medication, whether it has recently been changed, stopped or missed, may indicate further vulnerability.

18.4.1.10 Current mental state

A careful mental state, including whether or not there is current mental illness (which will both increase risk and will require intervention) and current thoughts about self-harm or suicide is essential (see Chapter 2).

18.4.1.11 A management plan

Ultimately, a decision about the best management plan for the patient in front of you will have to be made. At a junior level, your main role may be to ensure the patient is safe until someone more senior assesses the patient with you. This will include asking the patient if they have any immediate plans for self-harm, whether they feel 'safe' in the ED and (possibly) removing any immediate access to means. Often, you will also need to ensure the patient has someone with them (often termed a 'one to one special' nurse) until further assessment is possible.

These are all difficult decisions based on clinical judgement and you are likely to need senior advice.

If the person is being discharged home, they should be given a plan for their care. Ideally, a relative should be informed and aware, and a copy sent to the patient's GP. Finally, patients should be made aware of the various emergency access points available to them should they feel overwhelmed in the future.

18.5 Risk of harm to others

Clinical vignette Harm to others

'The man in the Emergency Department seemed manic—unable to sit still, shouting, laughing, with a constant stream of speech, joking to himself. He told me he had special powers given to him by God and he had to act to rid the world of people who were evil. He had specific plans and an idea of where he would start. He was angry that we suggested he might be ill and needed care, and were preventing him from carrying out his plan. He needed sedation, treatment, and admission under the Mental Health Act. I saw this man several weeks later in the psychiatry in-patient ward. He sat quietly throughout our interview, remembered our meeting in the Emergency Department. He was very distressed about his experiences, shocked and frightened that he had considered harming others.' Consultant Psychiatrist

Many of the factors relevant in the assessment of risk of self-harm also form part of the assessment of risk of harm to others (see Clinical vignette Harm to others). As in all situations, key is whether the person has a mental illness. Some individuals in the ED are threatening to harm others in the context of feuds, debts, or other issues. These are very different scenarios from a patient with a psychosis who is considering harming someone in the context of a delusional belief. Individuals who do not have mental illness will need to be referred to the appropriate agency, which may include the police. Again, discussion with senior colleagues is important, as there may be duties to inform others. Patients who are threatening to harm others in the context of acute mental illness will almost certainly require immediate admission for safety and to allow treatment of their illness. Again, discussion with senior colleagues and colleagues in the ED is very helpful in these complex cases (see also Chapter 15).

18.6 Other serious, high-risk adverse events

When interviewing patients, people may focus on risk of harm to self and others, and omit assessment of other risks that may be much more pertinent. The term 'risk' simply means the likelihood of some adverse event occurring.

Examples of other risks that may need to be clarified (and interventions considered when possible) include:

- Financial difficulties secondary to reckless spending or risk of financial exploitation by others (e.g. in mania).
- Loss of employment.
- Relationship breakdown.
- Harm due to impulsive behaviours, such as substance use or promiscuity, including physical injury, sexually transmitted diseases, or unwanted pregnancy.
- Impaired ability to care for children.

18.6.1 Medication-related emergencies

18.6.1.1 Neuroleptic malignant syndrome (NMS)

This is a rare, idiosyncratic, potentially fatal response to neuroleptic medication. It usually occurs shortly after starting, or increasing, doses. It is characterized clinically by:

- Fever.
- Rigidity (severe).
- Fluctuating levels of consciousness.
- Autonomic instability (fluctuating BP and HR).

Biochemically it is supported by the finding of grossly elevated creatine kinase.

There are several methods for diagnosis, including 'major' and 'minor' criteria. In its fully fledged presentation, it is a serious, potentially life-threatening condition with rhabdomyolysis, renal failure, seizures, and arrhythmias, requiring admission to intensive care. Management includes stopping antipsychotic medication and introduction of supportive and specific medical treatments, depending on the presentation and will require involvement of senior colleagues, often transfer to a medical unit.

Clinical problems associated with a diagnosis of NMS include:

- Difficulty in diagnosis in milder cases:
  - O Many patients on antipsychotics will have rigidity, may have pyrexia and tachycardia for other reasons (such as infection) and a moderately raised creatine kinase (CK) (if, for example, they have bruising due to a fall).
- A diagnosis of NMS carries significant implications for patient management, as it will require discontinuation of antipsychotic medication and slow, careful introduction of an alternative. This carries risks of relapse and deterioration in the patient's mental health and, therefore, must not be made lightly.

18.6.1.2 Serotonin syndrome

A clinical syndrome characterized by:

- Pyrexia.
- Agitation and confusion.
- Rigidity (mild), tremors, and hyperreflexia.
- Tachycardia and blood pressure instability.
- Occurs in the context of increased serotonergic activity:
  - O SSRIs, or an interaction between an SSRI and other agents that influence serotonin.
  - O Need a high index of suspicion in hospital where patients may already be on an SSRI and another apparently 'innocuous' agent is added, e.g. pain (opioid) medication, such as tramadol, or antibiotics (linezolid).
- Management includes:
  - O Stopping the serotonergic agent.
  - O Supportive medical care tailored to the presentation, e.g. hydration, benzodiazepines for agitation or seizures.

18.6.1.3 Lithium toxicity

Lithium is an extremely effective drug in the treatment of affective disorder. However:

- It is highly susceptible to **drug interactions and increased (toxic) levels**, largely due to narrow therapeutic window and because, like sodium, it is filtered and partly reabsorbed by the kidney, e.g. in dehydration, when the proximal tubule absorbs more water, lithium is also reabsorbed and levels rise. Similarly, because it is reabsorbed in competition with sodium, when sodium levels fall (e.g. with thiazide diuretics), lithium re-absorption increases.

- **NSAIDs, ACE inhibitors, and calcium channel-blockers** all may increase levels of lithium.
- Usual therapeutic range is 0.7–1.2 mmol/l (measured 12 h after the last dose).
- Early symptoms of toxicity may appear between 1.5 and 2.0 mmol/l, with serious toxicity at levels greater than 2.0 mmol/l.
- Tolerance to lithium may reduce with age.
- Symptoms of toxicity include tremor, anorexia, nausea, and vomiting, progressing to slurred speech, muscle twitching, ataxia, and confusion. This can rapidly progress to seizures and coma, and represents a medical emergency.
- Management includes stopping lithium, re-hydration, and transfer to medical care where treatment, including renal dialysis, may be needed. Symptoms of lithium toxicity often persist for some time after plasma levels have reduced.

18.7 Summary

There are many scenarios in psychiatry that present as urgent, serious, high-risk situations. These include clinical presentations with risk to self and others, acute behavioural disturbance (again with risk to self or others), and risk in the context of treatments. Some of these scenarios are unique to a mental health context, as it is rare for patients presenting to physicians and surgeons to be at risk of harming themselves or others. Assessing these scenarios presents specific challenges. As in any situation for students (and junior doctors), careful consideration of the factors involved, a thorough assessment, maximizing safety, and, most importantly, asking for the help and advice of a senior colleague and team members are key.

CHAPTER 19

Professionalism, boundaries, and well-being

'... Medicine is different from most other professions, not by virtue of its length of training, or the depth of knowledge, but by its code of behaviour and its concern with people ...'

James McCormick, Professor of Social Medicine
(later Community Health) at Trinity College,
Dublin (1973–91) in The Doctor: Father Figure or
Plumber (1979, p.13) Guilford, Surrey. Biddles Ltd.

CHAPTER FOCUS

What you should know about professionalism

- Be aware of the challenges and rewards of working in medicine.
- Understand the huge responsibilities that professionalism places on young students and doctors.
- The complex and far-reaching implications of being committed to confidentiality.
- The function of boundaries
- How to be kind to yourself, promoting self-care and resilience.

19.1 Introduction

This chapter focuses on the challenges and rewards of working in medicine. It discusses what is expected of us, suggests ways that we can protect and strengthen ourselves, enabling us to best look after our patients. It reminds us that, in preparing for a role of a life-time of caring for others, we would do well to first ensure that we have put in place strategies to look after ourselves.

19.2 Professionalism

19.2.1 What is professionalism?

While 'professionalism' is now at the centre of much discussion in medicine, and particularly in the field of medical education (Medical Council), the term itself only came to prominence in the 1980s. As is evident from the quote above, however, it has long been recognized that becoming a doctor brings with it responsibilities beyond the work itself, commitments to a code of behaviour, and service to others.

The practice of medicine requires knowledge, intellect, and skill, embedded in a set of beliefs and attitudes. It necessitates the integration of two strands: the 'service' aspects of medicine (work, maintenance of competence, autonomy, and self-regulation) together with humanism (an interest and concern for humanity) that requires commitment to caring, altruism, trust, respect, integrity, and confidentiality.

The American Board of Internal Medicine (ABIM) notes that doctors must demonstrate clinical competence, communication skills, ethical and legal knowledge, governed by commitment to excellence, integrity, empathy, respect, accountability, and altruism.

These descriptions allow some recognition not only of the complexity of the role of being a doctor, but also the far-reaching, personal demands that being a doctor brings. Many of these statements are personally challenging: the concept that one must put someone else's needs (usually a total stranger) above one's own (even when that may involve significant personal cost); that pursuit of financial rewards cannot be the main motivation (crucial if patients are not to be subjected to inappropriate tests, examinations, and reviews), that trust, truth, honesty, and integrity are core, even when that may be against the best interest of the self. These are challenging codes of behaviour to adopt. Add to that the need for doctors to be honest but not blunt, compassionate but not distressed, knowledgeable but not paternalistic, detached but not callous, to advise but not to control, (see Table 19.1), the task seems Herculean. Many of these codes of behaviour continue to be required beyond the workplace. The codes of conduct for the medical council mean that conviction for any offence will lead to suspension from the medical register. For young medical students, these are difficult concepts. Many are not even aware of them as they set off on their path. For students entering into the field of mental health, these requirements for honesty, integrity, and compassion, balanced with objectivity, are even more critical, as

Table 19.1 The impossible balance of roles for a doctor	
To be:	But not:
Honest	Blunt
Empathic	Distressed
Knowledgeable	Paternalistic
Objective	Callous
Advising	Controlling

the discipline entails working with particularly vulnerable people, discussing highly confidential, personal experiences.

19.2.2 What are the (personal) gains of professionalism?

It is important to remember that, as in many things in life, there are gains as well as costs. There are many wonderful experiences in being a doctor. Many of these are what drew students into medicine in the first place. And, in truth, these often only increase in magnitude with advancing years in training and service. There is a huge reward in knowing one has contributed to someone's life; satisfaction with a job well done; and the sense that one can make a real difference, sometimes by the smallest of tasks, often acknowledged directly by patients. However, this belief that one can make a difference, the responsibility of being entrusted with someone's care, brings with it necessary demands and costs that must be considered to allow young (and old) doctors to continue to perform well and to be well themselves (essential if they are to perform well).

19.2.3 What are the (personal) costs of professionalism?

Table 19.1 outlines a series of demands that are, at best, extremely challenging and, at worst, overwhelming. The requirement for doctors to 'know the answers', provide the solutions, care without being overwhelmed, and put others' needs before their own, is an enormous task. This is often worsened by the training experience. Medicine generally selects high-achievers—perfectionistic, conscientious individuals who strive for success. Furthermore, the emphasis on training is typically on 'knowing the answers', finding solutions. While this is clearly important, it needs to be balanced by a recognition that it is just not possible to have all the answers. Indeed, particularly in serious illnesses, there are no '**cures**', only a **commitment to care** for the person to the best of one's ability. Often described as the 'hidden curriculum', these issues, if not recognized and managed as actively as other areas of the curriculum, can lead to doctors becoming overwhelmed, distressed, and ultimately 'burnt-out' or ill.

The very values that make medicine so rewarding (believing one can make a difference, sense of being entrusted with care, knowledge one has impacted positively on someone's life), are what make it so difficult. When treatment fails, many clinicians describe a sense of grief, guilt, failure, exhaustion, frustration, futility—feelings that can increase over a career.

As with any problem, one of the first steps to address it, is to be aware of it, and then to provide intervention early, if possible, to prevent it. This means building awareness in student doctors to allow them to prepare for, and manage, the challenges from the beginning. The sections that follow discuss some of these concepts. There are no easy solutions. Even the concept of altruism, putting the patient's needs first (a central commitment for any other doctor), can become embroiled in controversy. How does one balance this with doctors' needs to have their own lives, their own commitments, and responsibilities to families, friends, themselves? (see Clinical vignette Professionalism; Figure 19.1).

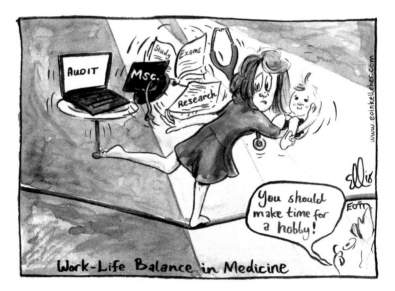

Figure 19.1 Professionalism—the 'tightrope' of the doctor in training.
© Eoin Kelleher.

Clinical vignette Professionalism

'I am very frustrated with everyone telling me to "look after myself", to find a "balance". How can I do that, when I rarely leave work before 7 p.m., must be in by 7.30 a.m., and frequently cancel meetings with friends at the last minute because of work. The concept that I should also have time to shop for nutritious food, cook and eat well, and have several hobbies, is just a joke. Added to that is the stress of being the most junior doctor on the team, desperate to do a good job, but frequently finding I do not know what to do next. Many patients I assess are my age, some have died. I often feel overwhelmed.' Junior Doctor

If these are not addressed, and a balance found, then there is the risk that we will continue to see a steady rise in physician ill-health and suffering. And, ironically but truthfully, this will ultimately impact not only their colleagues, but also the patients for whom they care. It is in the best interest of everyone—patients and staff alike—to address these issues.

19.3 Confidentiality

Ensuring that what patients have told you remains absolutely confidential to you (and relevant team members) is crucial and is one of the very first issues you will encounter, as you are handed the 'patient list' on your first day. When you start as a medical student, it can be difficult to realize just how important it is, and how challenging it can be, to ensure this. You must learn to never discuss patients outside the immediate medical environment. Avoid carrying any information relating to patients outside the hospital environment.

It is difficult sometimes to realize how difficult this can be. Any document or piece of paper you carry with patient information on it, is highly confidential. If you must carry it from one place (within the hospital) to another, you must make sure it is not visible to anyone else, and keep it with you at all times. You should not discuss patients' histories outside the clinical setting, or with other people (even close friends or colleagues). It would be a huge betrayal of patient trust for them to hear even part of their history relayed back through a third party. While these may seem like minor challenges, it requires self-discipline to refrain from discussing interesting cases with close colleagues or friends, unless in the interests of patient care. Equally, many students have experienced the overwhelming distress of finding they have misplaced a confidential letter or patient list. The vigilance and care required, even in this most minor of tasks, is significant (see Practical tips Students—how to avoid breaching confidentiality).

Practical tips Students—how to avoid breaching confidentiality

- **Never** discuss patients except in private, clinical environments.
- Do **not** carry around patient information unless absolutely necessary (printed hospital lists are particularly treacherous).
- Avoid using identifying names, initials, dates of birth, address, etc., again unless necessary.

The right of the patient to confidentiality is paramount but, as always in medicine, there are some situations where this is overridden. This includes any disclosure of child sexual abuse or where there is a risk of danger to the public or self. If you are uncertain, always discuss it with your team (see Chapter 1).

19.4 Boundaries

One of the challenges and privileges of working in mental health is that a significant amount of work is done through clinical interviewing and **personal interaction**—both assessment and treatment. For many people outside psychiatry this is seen as 'just talking' and 'what harm can it do?'. Given that the nature of the relationship between doctors and patients, particularly in mental health, is often long-standing and highly individualized, it is extremely important that clear, well-defined boundaries are in place, emphasizing that these are **professional not personal** relationships. While this is particularly important in psychiatry, it is relevant in all aspects of medicine.

19.4.1 How do boundaries work?

In everyday life, people are aware of physical boundaries: walls, hedges, doors, fences. People naturally understand what they are and how they function. Boundaries act to clearly demarcate areas, of (personal) space and safety. They are generally respected—usually their size and physical presence enforces them. Some 'physical' boundaries are not so obvious—'ground-lines' in sports or in a car-park. Although they are not a 'physical' block, they function because people recognize them as boundaries, understand the rules that govern them, and know that they will be penalized for failing to respect them. These boundaries provide safety, order, and clarity. While boundaries provide protection, they also carry with them responsibility—to function well they must be maintained. Furthermore, while usually helpful, boundaries can also do harm. Excessive boundaries run the risk of isolation; lack of adequate boundaries may draw trespass, abuse, or stigma.

Although rarely considered in this manner, these qualities of physical boundaries apply to **boundaries** that operate in **personal interactions** (see Table 19.2). Body space, gesture, touch, eye contact, rate and volume of speech, all serve as 'boundaries' in personal interactions that give messages about an interaction. Caring, considerate, bored, angry, threatening, dismissive—these are all messages that can be given very clearly without ever having to verbalize the message. Every student can recount having observed these interactions. This may be the intention of the communicator, a scenario for which they must take responsibility. Sometimes, however, the behaviour is unconscious, and the message transmitted inadvertently. Being aware of all our communication strategies is the first step to ensure that we transmit to others that which we wish to transmit.

For doctors working in mental health, the content and context of the interview are often highly personal. Potentially sensitive and intimate information is

Table 19.2 Psychological boundaries—some examples

Non-verbal (implied)	Verbal (implied)	Specified
Dress (attire)—formal or informal	Tone	Use of patient's first-name
Inter-personal space	Speed of speech	Use of own first-name
Eye contact	Number of pauses	Environment
Posture/gestures	Brevity (monosyllabic)	Personal effects on display (or not)
Non-verbal (direct)	**Verbal (stated/direct)**	Office-style
Touch	I have plenty of time	
Hug	I don't have time for questions	

discussed that would normally only be shared in the context of close, personal relationships. The message given about boundaries for the interaction must be that it is a caring, empathic, respectful, and, above all, a **professional interaction**; one that is safe for the patient and safe for the doctor. This requires a careful setting-up of the interaction from the very beginning to ensure that it is clearly distinguishable from an interaction with a close, personal confidante. Each student (and doctor) will have to decide for themselves what types of boundaries they are comfortable with as, much as with houses, people will differ in their 'styles'. One of the first decisions will be **how to address the patient**, for example. This may be more formally—Mr X or Ms Y, or by first-name terms. Similar rules apply to how one introduces oneself. A more formal introduction helps to clarify that it is a professional not a personal relationship. Age and culture will affect this. Asking the patient how they would like to be addressed is helpful, or they may volunteer themselves (or correct you). The **physical environment** must also be considered (see Chapter 1). Doctors must also decide how much of their **personal lives** they share with patients. Again, people differ. Some suggest that display of personal items shows they are willing to share and engage with the patient, that they are more 'human'. Others suggest doctors should be able to do this without the need to display personal items and that there is a risk of causing offence/distress or impeding the patient's ability to confide, if items are on view that are contrary to their beliefs. Perhaps the **key issue** here is that doctors (and student doctors) **actively consider these concepts** and make decisions based on their views, rather than finding they have 'wandered' into situations they then find very difficult to amend (see Clinical vignette Boundaries). Certainly, the medical councils governing doctors' behaviour in many countries specifically cite the importance of maintaining professional boundaries, and warn against the risks of blurring boundaries between personal and professional lives, particularly with the increasing use of social media.

Clinical vignette Boundaries

'My first post as a junior doctor was as an oncology trainee. My first patient was my age, from near my home-town in rural Ireland. I had never considered how I would balance my personal and professional interactions. He was a charming, kind, young man who never complained, despite a horrific illness and dreadful side-effects of treatment. And, after seeing him daily for four months as an in-patient, getting to know his parents, brothers, and sisters, he died. Thirty years on, I still remember. I was totally unprepared for the impact of his death. The case was a hard, but valuable, learning point for me. I realized I could not get as personally involved with every patient—I would never survive a career in oncology. I had to remember my own life, while caring for patients as well as I possibly could. I also recognized that I had to be fair, to treat all patients equally, even those with whom I could not so easily identify. That is the challenge.' Oncologist

19.4.2 The role of boundaries for patients and clinicians

A clear definition between personal and professional roles for patients helps to protect against:

- Patients having unrealistic expectations.
- Inappropriate relationships with vulnerable patients.
- Lack of balance in interactions with patients (the 'lovely' versus the 'challenging' patient).
- Undermining of other staff by 'special' relationships with patients.
- Personal values interfering with professional judgement.
- Professionals becoming over-involved on a personal level.

19.5 Setting limits

One of the central concepts in professionalism is altruism, the concept of putting patients' needs first. This does not mean, however, that students or doctors must respond and comply with every request. Sometimes the role of the doctor (particularly in mental health) is to provide safe, clear limits as to what can, and will, be tolerated. This must be done in a compassionate, measured, and clear manner. For some patients, this concept of **containment**—that the doctor can manage and contain challenging behaviour—can be a very helpful learning experience. Equally, no person should accept abuse—physical or verbal.

A broader aspect of setting limits is for young doctors and medical students to be aware of their own limits—professional and personal. Much of medical school is focused on the concept that medical students must know the answer for every question (it is generally what they pass and fail their exams on). However, it is not possible to always know the answer and an important lesson is to know your professional limits, to let the patient know you do not know the answer and to **ask for help,** particularly from senior colleagues. It is inevitable that you will make a mistake. One cannot be human without making one.

Setting limits with family and friends in your new role as a doctor can present unexpected challenges. You may find yourself the recipient of many requests— for medical opinions, psychiatric opinions, even medical prescriptions. You must learn to listen to your instincts and consider your professional duties (see Clinical vignette Setting limits).

Clinical vignette Setting limits

"I was the first doctor in our family—in fact the first doctor from our rural village. Everyone was very proud. Six months after qualifying, I had a phone-call from my aunt. She was due to fly on holiday the next day. Terrified of flying, she "knew" that "Valium" would help her, and, now that I was a doctor, I could prescribe it. I was

continued >

---

particularly close to this aunt, who had supported me during difficult times. It was so tempting to write a prescription, to "help"—and so very difficult to say "no". Conflicting emotions—wanting to help, sense of loyalty, duty, and affection for my aunt, fighting with a sense of discomfort at writing a prescription I knew was not appropriate, and awareness of ethical obligations. I could hear her disappointment and anger when I said no—my first experience of trying to keep a limit between my personal and professional life. Over the years, I learned to recognize those feelings, and listen to them. It does not mean one cannot help—general advice, often recommending contact with their own GP, and supportive listening, are always available. But one must stay within one's professional boundaries.' Physician

With respect to **personal limits**, safe-guarding areas outside medicine is crucial. Medicine is often all-consuming. Setting goals to limit work to the work-space, to prioritize meeting friends (especially those 'outside' medicine), and to maintain talents or interests you have is key, even though it can seem an impossible task (Figure 19.1). Fortunately, recently, there has been a more widespread acceptance of the importance of these concepts of self-care.

19.6 Self-care and resilience

19.6.1 What is resilience?

Although there is no single agreed definition of resilience, the basic elements refer to an ability to 'bounce back' in the face of adversity, to adapt and respond to challenges and stress. This ability varies within and between individuals, with age, and with the nature of the challenge. Factors thought to promote resilience include supportive relationships, a positive view of one's abilities, skills in problem-solving and communication, an ability to manage strong feelings, to plan, and carry out, realistic solutions. Experiencing adverse events, provided they are not overwhelming, can help to strengthen future coping strategies—the caveat, *that they are not overwhelming*, is particularly important. A reliable support network and approachable, supportive senior colleagues are among the factors that can help to ensure this.

It would not be possible to eliminate all stressors from the work of junior hospital doctors. Daily, you will experience a large range of events, from relatively minor incidents, to major ones that may involve, for example, the sudden and unexpected death of patients for whom you feel responsible. When you first qualify, these are often shocking, remaining in your memory for years afterwards (see Clinical vignette Boundaries). However, learning to manage this is essential to ensure you can continue to work. As discussed above, previous exposure to stressful experiences can help to bolster responses to new events. A key factor, however, must be that these experiences should serve to promote a sense of self-efficacy, not be overwhelming. Events that promote a capacity for self-reflection, sense of control, sense of self-efficacy, and a sense of belonging to a community are important in this process. Supportive relationships with colleagues are key. An ability to seek help and learn from challenging (or successful) situations will naturally develop from these relationships, fostering opportunities to reflect on events and recognize what has gone well, or what needs to change. Echoing earlier chapters, working within a well-functioning MDT is a natural environment for this to occur. It can be difficult for junior doctors who are grappling with new environments, new roles, and new tasks, as well as new colleagues and team-mates, on a regular basis—ask for help.

Maintaining involvement in activities **outside work** (such as music or sport), particularly including a sense of community and involvement with others, is important.

The Royal College of Physicians in Ireland recommends a 'healthy mind platter', including physical activity, 'down-time', 'playtime', a focus on the here-and-now, and **social connection**. The medical council now includes **responsibility for self-care** as part of professionalism. This has put self-care as a central part of being a doctor, requiring a careful balance of the competing demands discussed above. Inevitably, caring for yourself will, in turn, result in better care for patients, and better environments for you, and everyone else, at work (Practical Tips Professionalism and self-care).

19.6.2 Resilience—a word of caution

Many of these concepts are considered within the theme of 'resilience', a concept that is, generally, to be applauded. However, there is a risk that promoting resilience suggests the 'blame' lies with those who are not 'tough' enough; it allows the 'system' to continue to place excessive demands on doctors with insufficient resources. This is not what resilience is about. Resilience is about promoting well-being, self-care, and self-efficacy to allow individuals to be as well as they possibly can when challenges come their way. And in the field of medicine, it is inevitable that those challenges will come, early and often, in medical careers. Clearly, also, the system and the environment must also be addressed (Figure 19.1). While we seek to provide interventions that allow doctors to function in difficult circumstances, we must never cease to seek other interventions to improve physician well-being, which includes reducing, or removing, stressors where possible.

Practical tips Professionalism and self-care

'K.L.A.S.H.'—'E.A.R.L.Y.' (and often):

- Be Kind—to yourself and others.
- Know your Limits (knowledge and boundaries).
- Attend to yourself with a HI Five:
  - Hobbies.
  - Interests.
  - Friendships.
- Prioritize Social networks—professional and personal.

continued >

- Ask for Help (shows strength, self-awareness, and a willingness to learn from others).

E.A.R.L.(Y):

- Be Empathic—(for yourself, patients, and team-mates).
- Accept that neither you, nor anyone else, is perfect.
- Respect those that you meet (and expect respect in turn).
- Learn from/reflect on your experiences—use this for the next time.

19.7 Summary

The principles that motivate doctors and are reinforced in medical training (striving for excellence, a huge commitment to service, compassion, and a desire to cure and to find solutions) are the very concepts that can prove overwhelming in their demands over time. The knowledge that one has helped others is a powerful reward. When, however, this commitment becomes all-consuming and prevents physicians from looking after themselves (and their families), it can lead to fatigue and burnout.

One of the difficulties is that consideration of these concepts, has, up to now, rarely been included within a medical curriculum. We hope, by bringing attention to them in this handbook, that it will provide an impetus for student doctors to reflect on these important concepts **early in their career**, considering boundaries and limits, fostering connections and supportive relationships from the start, maintaining interests and friendships outside, as well as inside, medicine.

Glossary

Affect Emotional state at a particular point in time, or in response to a particular event (shorter-lived than mood). Categories include: reactive (to interviewer); restricted (reduced, e.g. depression); labile (changes rapidly, e.g. mania, stroke); blunted (lacks emotional response, e.g. schizophrenia); congruent (appropriate) or incongruent (inappropriate) to situation.

Akathisia Distressing feeling of inner restlessness with an overwhelming need to keep moving. Often a side-effect of medication.

Alexithymia Difficulty recognizing and expressing emotions and empathizing with others. Not linked with a particular diagnosis, associated with somatization disorders.

Amnesia Partial or total (global) inability to recall past events. May be psychological, e.g. dissociative amnesia (at times of great stress) or physical, e.g. Korsakoff's syndrome.

Anhedonia Unable to feel any pleasure or enjoyment (key symptom of depression)

Apathy Extreme lack of emotional response, activity and sense of futility. Particularly associated with hopelessness, adverse circumstances, negative symptom of schizophrenia.

Athetosis Involuntary, continuous writhing (twisting) movements, usually of the hands or feet. Seen in cerebral palsy or post-stroke.

Auditory Hallucinations See hallucinations.

Automatic Obedience Does whatever is requested, regardless of consequences (severe schizophrenia).

Catalepsy/Waxy Flexibility Allows limbs to be moved into any position, hold this position for prolonged period, even after pressure has been removed (cf. mitmachen/mitgehen when returns to their normal resting position) (severe schizophrenia).

Catatonia Ambiguous term, specifically refers to particular motor signs (waxy flexibility and echopraxia [see entries]) with disorders of thought, mood, or behaviour. More frequently, non-specific severe, prolonged features (agitation or withdrawal). Occurs in schizophrenia, mania, depression, and several medical conditions.

Charles Bonnet Syndrome Vivid visual hallucinations but no other features of either mental or physical illness, usually in older people with visual impairment; disappear once eyesight has improved or with total loss of vision.

Chorea/Choreiform Movements Sudden, involuntary muscle spasms, typically non-goal directed. Often hidden by turning them into a voluntary gesture. Occurs in neurological conditions (Huntington's disease—mainly in upper body).

Circumstantiality Painstaking, excessive, unnecessary detail but lacks the vividness of detail of 'flight of ideas' (see Flight of Ideas entry). Eventually reaches a conclusion Associated with obsessional personality traits, or anxiety, but not diagnostic of any specific disorder.

Clang Associations Person connects words because they sound the same (mania), e.g. 'Dr Dunne, that's done it'.

Command Hallucination The person hears a voice or voices telling them to do something, may or may not feel compelled to act on this.

Compulsion Behaviour (action or thought) the person feels compelled to do; usually to prevent a negative outcome, though acknowledges there is no logical connection between feared outcome and the behaviour. Does not enjoy it. Specific, ritualized pattern to behaviour. Examples: excessive handwashing or checking behaviours. Feature of obsessive–compulsive disorder.

Confabulation Plausible but false memories to fill memory gaps. Seen in organic/physical causes of amnesia such as Korsakoff's. NOT deliberate attempt to mislead.

Déjà-vu Non-specific, vague sense that something being experienced for the first time has been experienced before. Part of normal experience, also temporal lobe epilepsy, schizophrenia.

Delusion Fixed false belief, held with absolute certainty despite evidence to the contrary, not in keeping with the person's cultural or religious beliefs, often bizarre in nature.

Depersonalisation/Derealization Complex concept, unpleasant sensation of being 'cut off'/distant from emotions; person feels as if they are not real. Often also feel as if environment is unreal (derealisation). Occurs in many settings (sleep deprivation, severe stress, mental illness). Not delusional experiences (retains insight).

Derailment No meaningful connection between thoughts (schizophrenia).

Dissociation (of affect) Marked reduction in appropriate fear or anxiety. Several forms: 'denial' (usually fluctuates) where person seems not to understand, believe, or accept what is happening (e.g. diagnosis of cancer), while still, for example, attending for chemotherapy; 'belle indifference', seen in hysteria where patients are completely undisturbed by severe disability.

Dysarthria Difficulty with articulation or physical production of speech. Due to local (pharynx or tongue) or central (brainstem) lesions. Still understands and writes without impairment.

Dysphasia Difficulty with language, expression (expressive) or understanding (receptive). Due to central (brain) lesions: Broca's area (dominant frontal lobe) results in expressive (non-fluent) (Broca's) dysphasia; Wernicke's area (left temporal lobe) results in a receptive (Wernicke's) dysphasia. (Aphasia = complete loss of language).

Dystonia Abrupt, involuntary contraction of any muscle group. Side-effect of medication (esp. anti-psychotic).

Echolalia Repeats words/phrases spoken by others. Seen in schizophrenia, learning disability, dementia.

Echopraxia Repeats the actions or gestures of others.

Elemental Hallucinations SImple hallucinations (flashes of light or noises) rather than fully formed images. Typical of organic (physical) conditions, e.g. delirium.

Euphoria Excessive cheerfulness (seen in mania, frontal lobe damage),

Flight of Ideas Ideas 'jump', rapidly, and apparently randomly, from one topic to the next; thought connections can be difficult to discern, are often simply due to outside distractions, or chance and may be associated with words that rhyme (clang associations) ('red, read, I read it there') or through the use of puns (punning) (mania).

Formal Thought Disorder Disorder of form/structure of thoughts.

Formication Tactile hallucination—sensation of insects crawling over the body (seen with cocaine abuse).

Hallucination Perception in the absence of an external stimulus (to its related sensory organ). Experienced as real, occur in external space, not under voluntary control. Can occur in each of the sensory modalities: auditory, visual, gustatory (taste), olfactory (smell), somatic (bodily sensations), tactile (touch). Usually, auditory hallucinations suggest a primary mental illness and visual hallucinations suggest organic (physical) brain disease, such as delirium.

Hyperaesthesia Sensations seem more intense, e.g. more sensitive to sounds (hyperacusis) (migraine); colours more vivid (LSD or mania).

Hyperamnesia An event remembered with exaggerated clarity and detail, usually associated with strong emotion, e.g. the 'flashbacks' of post-traumatic stress disorder, or use of hallucinogens.

Hypnagogic and Hypnopompic Hallucinations Normal experience, not diagnostic of mental illness. False perceptions that occur while falling asleep (hypnagogic) or waking up (hypnopompic). They can be auditory, visual or tactile. Hypnagogic hallucinations are much more common and happen when the person is drowsy; usually auditory, e.g. hearing a knock on the door or someone calling your name (when it hasn't really happened). The person may believe that they were wide awake at the time but studies have disproved this.

Hypoaesthesia Sensations less intense, e.g. in delirium, depression.

Illusion Misinterpretation of a stimulus, e.g. thinks shadow of hedge on dark road is an attacker; worse with heightened emotion or reduced stimuli. Also occurs when brain 'imagines' objects are present to make sense of images.

Insight Person's understanding of their illness, not an all or nothing phenomenon, fluctuates. Components include: belief there is something wrong; due to illness (mental or physical); treatment available that will help them and that they accept.

Jamais-vu Sense places are unfamiliar even though experienced before; part of everyday experience, schizophrenia, temporal lobe epilepsy.

Lilliputian Hallucinations Visual hallucinations of tiny people, animals, or objects associated with severe alcohol withdrawal.

Micropsia/Macropsia Objects are perceived as smaller/larger than they really are (due to visual problems or damage to the temporal or parietal lobes).

Mitgehen ('angle-poise lamp sign') Exaggerated form of mitmachen (person moves in response to slightest pressure despite instructions to resist).

Mitmachen Allow their body to be moved into any position despite instructions to resist, slowly return to resting position.

Mood A person's emotional state over a prolonged period of time, defines the person's experience. Can be depressed (low); elated/manic (high) or 'normothymic' ('normal').

Mutism Does not speak but fully conscious. Occurs in several situations, e.g. learning disability, organic brain disorders, catatonic schizophrenia, depressive illnesses Elective mutism (children), refuse to speak in certain situations.

Negativism Needlessly resists all instructions: passive (simply do nothing in response to instruction) or active (do the opposite of instruction).

Neologisms Invents words or gives existing words new, unique meaning (schizophrenia). Different from expressive dysphasia where word used incorrectly.

Obsessions Repetitive, intrusive, unwanted thoughts, images, or impulses that the person tries to resist. Content distressing and typically repugnant to the person, e.g. violent thoughts, images, or impulses in a quiet, timid person; sexual content in a person by nature prudish; blasphemy in someone with strong religious beliefs. Person recognizes them as their own ('home-made but disowned'), differentiating this from thought insertion (see Thought Insertion entry).

Over-Valued Idea Intensely held belief, not of delusional intensity, usually associated with intense feeling and dominates the person's life. Can occur in the absence of mental illness; can be difficult to distinguish from delusion.

Parkinsonism Symptoms similar to Parkinson's disease (shuffling gait, tremor muscular rigidity). Medication-related (antipsychotics).

Passivity Phenomena (Delusions of Control) Believes their emotions/impulses/actions/bodily sensations are under the control of an external agency or force. Sometimes termed 'made' emotions/impulses/actions/somatic passivity, respectively.

Pathological Emotionalism Intense outbursts of uncontrollable emotion (laughter or crying) often at inappropriate times causing distress and embarrassment. Milder form (lability of affect) refers to rapid changes in emotion (switching from tears to laughter, or easily being moved to tears or laughter), associated with organic/physical brain disease.

Perseveration The person senselessly repeats their actions (behaviour or speech) even when it no longer makes sense (catatonia and in organic/physical brain disease).

Poverty of Speech (Alogia) Reduction in the rate, volume, and spontaneity of speech. Reflects poverty of thought (severe depressive illnesses, chronic schizophrenia).

Poverty of Thought Reduction in rate and volume of thoughts (severe depression).

Pressure of Speech Increased rate (and often volume) of speech. Typical of mania (usually very difficult to interrupt). Also in anxiety but easy to interrupt.

Pseudologica Fantastica (Pathological Lying) False account (usually dramatic) of past events. Antisocial or hysterical personality disorders, particularly when stressed. When confronted with proof, the person often admits the lie.

Psychological Pillow Holds head just off the pillow—can hold this position for hours.

Psychomotor Agitation Restless, may be distressed (not specific to any one disorder, may be seen without mental illness when under stress).

Psychomotor Retardation Movements, thoughts, speech significantly slowed (typically seen in severe depression).

Recovered Memory Controversial phenomenon, particularly associated with recovered memories of childhood sexual abuse (CSA). Two viewpoints: that traumatic memories may be 'remembered' as an adult and are true, or, that the so-called 'memories' of abuse have been implanted during therapy by the power of suggestion.

Running Commentary Third-person auditory hallucinations, where voices are commenting on, discussing the person in the third person.

Schizophasia ('Word Salad', 'Verbigeration') Rare. Thoughts so disordered that they lack any meaning. Reflects severe disorder of thought form (schizophrenia).

Schneiderian First-Rank Symptoms of Scizophrenia Group of symptoms Schneider suggested were of the 'first-rank' and diagnostic of the schizophrenia. Include thought alienation, commentatory voices, and delusional perception. While not diagnostic (they can occur in other conditions, e.g. mania), the presence of these symptoms is highly suggestive of schizophrenia.

Stupor Mute, unresponsive state but seems fully conscious (may follow stimuli with their eyes). Can occur in severe depression, schizophrenia, or with frontal lobe or basal ganglia lesions.

Tardive Dyskinesia Involuntary, repetitive movements (grimacing, tongue protrusion, choreiform movements of the limbs or torso). Medication related (long-term use of older antipsychotics), often irreversible (unlike other side-effects).

Thought Alienation Combination of delusions of thought insertion, withdrawal, block, i.e. belief by the patient that their thoughts are not under their own control.

Thought Block/Stopping/Snapping Off Patient experiences sudden break in train of thought ('mind goes blank'). Occurs in schizophrenia. Often misinterpreted in a delusional way as due to an 'external force removing the thoughts from their head' (thought withdrawal).

Thought Broadcast Believes their thoughts are known to/can be read or heard by others—even strangers many miles away.

Thought Echo The person hears their thoughts being spoken out loud just before or just as they are formed (Gedankenlautwerden); thoughts are heard aloud just after they have formed (*echo de la pensée*).

Thought Insertion Believes some external force or agency is putting thoughts into their head.

Thought Withdrawal Believes some external force or agency is taking thoughts out of their head. (This may be the person's explanation for the phenomenon of thought block—see Thought Block/Stopping/Snapping Off entry.)

Tics—Motor, Vocal Sudden, repetitive movements (typically in face, e.g. blinking or movements of the forehead, nose or mouth) or vocalizations (simple noises, e.g. clearing of the throat, or complex words).

Vorbeireden (Talking Past the Point) 'Approximate answers.' Responds to questions with (almost correct) answer that shows they understood the question, e.g. when asked what colour is grass, answer 'white' (hysteria or pseudodementia). Also described by Ganser in criminals awaiting trial (Ganser syndrome).

Index

Please note that page references to Figures will be followed by the letter 'f', to Tables by the letter 't'